Advance Praise

"Sameera Khan is an incredibly knowledgeable guide on your weight loss journey following bariatric surgery. With decades of experience as a dietitian and physician assistant working with weight loss surgery patients, she is an invaluable resource. Her real-world tips are simple, but backed by science. The stories of the patients she has helped are inspiring. The excellent advice offered in this comprehensive book is reinforced by meaningful and useful graphics. As a bariatric surgeon, I plan to recommend this book to all my patients who are struggling to lose weight. Thank you to Ms. Khan for writing such a comprehensive resource".

Allison M. Barrett MD FACS FASMBS
Director of Bariatric Surgery at Penn State St. Joseph Medical Center
in Reading, Pennsylvania;
Clinical Assistant Professor of Surgery at Penn State University

"This book is an invaluable resource for patients and caregivers alike as it addresses the physical, emotional, psychological, and biochemical aspects of weight gain and weight regain. It is written in an extremely patient-friendly format with guidance, advice, and (most of all) excellent tools of empowerment for all readers."

Teresa R. Fraker, MS, RN
Program Administrator, MBSAQIP
American College of Surgeons

"This is the book I have been waiting for! It is a comprehensive review of the vexing problem of weight regain after bariatric surgery and is filled with wonderful insights for providers, patients and their loved ones. I have already started using some of the ideas and illustrations in my practice. It should be required reading for anyone interested in helping bariatric patients truly be successful in the long term."

Timothée Friesen, MD FACS
Bariatric and General Surgeon
Comprehensive Obesity Management Program
Greater Baltimore Medical Center, Baltimore, Maryland

"A huge thank you to the author for providing weight-loss surgery patients and their providers with such a wonderful tool! Ms. Khan's extensive experience working with patients and her passion for leading them to success to reach and maintain their goal is evident. This book is not only well written, filled with useful strategies, and backed by medical science, it is much needed in the bariatric specialty. I think the book has great application and can see it as excellent curriculum for use in support groups. I am grateful to have this useful book in my toolbox"!

Lynne Thompson, RN, CBN
Ex Vice President, Clinical Quality and Compliance
for the ASMBS Bariatric Surgery Center of Excellence Program
President, Lynne Thompson Consulting

"A great book and really good, comprehensive companion for both patients and practitioners."

William S. Richardson, MD, FACS, FAMBS
Professor, University of Queensland
Section Head General Surgery, Ochsner Clinic,
New Orleans, LA

"Regain Be Gone" is the first book I have read that pin points the problems and issues faced by real life bariatric patients in maintaining their goal weight after bariatric surgery. It is reader friendly with numerous illustrations and infographics that hold the interest of the person reading it. In addition to emphasizing the importance of sticking to doable protocols for long term weight loss it also guides the reader on how exactly to do it. In *Regain Be Gone* Khan explains in clear accessible language, what obstacles are encountered after bariatric surgery and what we can do to reverse it. This is a must read for health care professionals, and patients alike. As a physician who has also undergone bariatric surgery, this is the perfect resource for me and my bariatric patients on the go."

Farzin Sehati, DO
Internal Medicine Specialist

"Khan has written a comprehensive guide for all patients and providers. The combination of evidence based medicine and her extensive experience working with patients makes this one of the premier guides that every patient and provider should have on hand."

Cynthia J Inkpen, DHA, MPA, MA

"Sameera Khan is in her own lane with this fabulous book; She has removed all the roadblocks and barriers to achieve long term success for bariatric patients. Bravo"!

Kelly Mattone, MD
Physical Medicine & Rehabilitation

"This is not a diet book. Instead it describes a way of strategizing and overcoming the barriers weight loss surgery patients face years after surgery. Khan combines nutritional expertise and cutting edge principles into achievable strategies that any bariatric patient can follow."

Maria E. Peña, MD
Endocrinologist and Obesity Medicine Specialist
Mount Sinai Forest Hills Doctors
Director of Endocrine Services

"Obesity is an epidemic and an unrealized medical problem in the USA. Though there are medical and dietary treatments, long term, there has been poor success. Bariatric surgery has been shown to provide long term benefits and a great deal of improvement in medical health. After surgery, there are still problems adjusting to the drastic change in lifestyle. Ms. Khan's book walks you through the many obstacles involved and guides you to long term success. I highly recommend anyone who needs help in breaking a weight plateau after bariatric surgery to read this book."

Stuart Morduchowitz M.D.
Endocrinologist, Diabetes and Metabolism Specialist

Regain Be Gone

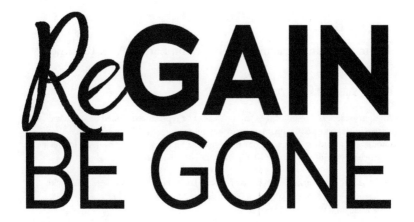

ReGAIN BE GONE

12 Strategies on Reclaiming the Body You Earned After Bariatric Surgery

SAMEERA KHAN, RD, PA-C

NEW YORK

LONDON • NASHVILLE • MELBOURNE • VANCOUVER

Regain Be Gone

12 Strategies on Reclaiming the Body You Earned After Bariatric Surgery

Published in New York, New York, by Morgan James Publishing in partnership with Difference Press. Morgan James is a trademark of Morgan James, LLC. www.MorganJamesPublishing.com

ISBN 9781642795837 paperback
ISBN 9781642795844 eBook
ISBN 9781642795851 audiobook
Library of Congress Control Number: 2019939509

Cover & Interior Design by:
Christopher Kirk
www.GFSstudio.com

Photography by:
Roza Siedlecki

This book is not intended as a substitute for the medical advice of surgeons or physicians. The reader should regularly consult a surgeon/physician in matters relating to his/her health, and particularly with respect to any symptoms that may require diagnosis or medical attention. This book is best paired as a supplemental resource to your bariatric post-op care team.

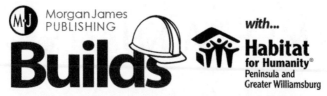

Morgan James is a proud partner of Habitat for Humanity Peninsula and Greater Williamsburg. Partners in building since 2006.

Get involved today! Visit
MorganJamesPublishing.com/giving-back

To all bariatric surgery patients who think I am writing about them…

I am.

Table of Contents

Foreword

Over the span of my career as a bariatric surgeon, a lot has changed. Surgery is now much safer, and can be applied to much sicker patients with outstanding results. I have witnessed amazing weight loss achievements in most of my patients as well as significant weight loss regains. The one thing that hasn't changed significantly and is the source of frustration for both patient and health care provider, is weight regain following surgery. Success depends primarily on the individual patient, their motivation, and their drive.

Despite improvement in health and wellbeing for most patients undergoing weight loss surgery, whether it is restrictive, malabsorptive, or both, weight regain to some degree is experienced by most, if not all, patients.

The degree, however, is what differs. Approximately 20-30% of patients will return to the pre-surgery status. For some, their comorbid medical conditions will return. For some, weight regain was the result they sub-consciously were looking for due to the difficulties of lifetime adherence, or a real lack of understanding of the post weight loss surgery lifestyle. For most dedicated compliant patients 10-20% weight regain above their lowest postoperative weight is common, and can be problematic.

To be successful, you must make long lasting changes in your post-operative bariatric life by watching portion sizes, eating the right amount of carbs, and consistently following an exercise program that you enjoy. The way you lose weight after weight loss surgery determines how you are going to be able to keep it off over the long run. Success is fostered by accountability and cognitively monitoring what you eat and how you exercise way past the "honeymoon" period.

This book is meant for those patients who are struggling to overcome the barriers that arise after bariatric surgery. The hope is it will provide an easy-to-follow resource tool for all of you who struggle with the same ten to fifteen pounds, to prevent it from becoming twenty five or thirty pounds.

The strategies and observations to follow come from real life patients with whom Sameera Khan has worked and has helped to prevent weight regain. It will hopefully serve to help you with your lifetime bariatric journey, or the journey of your patients.

Good luck on your weight loss journey!

Dr. Dominick Gadaleta, MD, FACS, FASMBS
Associate Professor of Surgery,
Donald and Barbara Zucker School of Medicine at Hofstra/ Northwell
Chair of Surgery, Southside Hospital, Chief of General Surgery,
Director of Metabolic and Bariatric and Robotic Surgery,
North Shore University Hospital

Sameera Khan has worked for years with my patients, helping them lose weight and keep it off after bariatric surgery. Although there is significant emphasis on the surgical aspect of this journey, we have learned over the past twenty years that without behavioral and nutritional changes, the success rate for optimal weight loss is not as good as it could be.

My patients are very happy, satisfied, and on the path to lifelong weight loss goals after working with Sameera. She absolutely gets results.

I began to refer my bariatric patients to her on a regular basis. When my patients return to their follow-up appointments, they are constantly saying how positive and important her guidance is to their weight loss. I have seen excellent patient compliance with the nutritional aspect of their weight loss journey.

Sameera has a great knowledge of how the body works after bariatric surgery. She works with patients in an easy and pleasant manner. She provides a light at the end of the "bariatric journey" despair. My patients are so fond of her and are motivated and inspired by her. I wish everyone who had bariatric surgery could meet someone like Sameera personally, but know it's impossible. That's why I am so happy she wrote this book which will serve as an invaluable resource for bariatric patients during their weight loss journey, or for those patients who are struggling to get back on track. I've seen Sameera help my patients. I can't wait to give a copy of this book to every struggling patient of mine.

It reiterates most of the reasons and saboteurs that result in regaining weight after bariatric surgery, and shows how to tackle them head on.

The fact that you have picked this book off the bookshelf is a great sign that you are ready to overcome any barriers you have encountered after bariatric surgery.

Wishing you all the success on reaching your post-surgery weight loss goals.

Congratulations! With Sameera Khan's help, you and your post - bariatric body are about to start healing.

Larry Gellman, MD, FACS, FASMBS
Chief Division of Minimally Invasive Surgery
Co-Director of Bariatric Surgery
North Shore University Hospital

Perspectives from Bariatric Surgeons

A Bariatric Surgeon's Perspective of Weight Regain after Surgery
by Larry Gellman, MD

Weight loss surgery is a very powerful treatment for obesity, but it is possible for patients to regain some or all the weight they have lost. There could be many reasons for this. Plateauing or regaining weight after the patient has gone through these procedures can be very distressing to the patient. Almost all patients will lose weight in the initial period following surgery, whether that is a lap-band, a gastric bypass, a sleeve gastrectomy, or many of the other procedures available. Sometimes this is referred to as the "honeymoon period." Why patients regain weight, how they regain weight, and what can be done about this has been a difficult problem. There have been many improvements in bariatric surgery over the years. Improvements in the actual procedures, preoperative preparation, and postoperative care have led to a decrease in morbidity and mortality, as well as increasing success long-term. There have been many opinions regarding all of this, but what we can all agree upon is that a team approach is critical, and that surgery for these selected patients is, and will continue to be, the gold standard for significant weight loss now and in the future. We must continue to stress that surgery is only the beginning of a long and successful journey. Destructive behaviors have led the patient to become morbidly obese. This will continue to be the most important long-term issue facing the patient and the clinicians charged with taking care of them.

Weight loss surgery is not a "miracle" but a "tool" that can be worked efficiently by the patient to reach their weight loss goals. Successful patients understand and realize this in addressing their bad habits and issues, all which led them to having weight loss surgery in the first place.

Some positive aids I have seen help my patients are:
- Having a supportive system

- Preparing for success with a planned schedule
- Developing social relationships with people who are active
- Educating themselves about nutrition, psychological issues, pitfalls, and physical activity
- Getting the right help with transfer of addictions

Patients need to recognize and own up to the lifestyle choices and issues that got them to sit across the chair from me considering weight loss surgery. If not, these issues will not change into better habits after surgery, and they will not be successful in keeping the weight off long term.

Change is hard. I see patients get frustrated and falling off track when they regain weight. If they do not show up to support groups, start taking accountability for themselves, or stay away from the surgical team, it spells disaster.

I expect my successful patients to get it right 80% of the time. One bad meal or one day of not exercising in no way sabotages your weight loss. It's the weeks of not eating right and not exercising before and after that one day that make them regain all their weight after bariatric surgery.

Weight loss surgery is a "second chance" given to obese patients, to reboot their "set point." The question is: Do patients realize the opportunity before them that will help them live healthier lives and negotiate pitfalls, or do they return to the point of no return?

Larry Gellman. MD, FACS, FASMBS
Chief of Minimally Invasive Surgery
Co-Director Bariatric Surgery
North Shore University Hospital

A Bariatric Surgeon's Perspective of Weight Regain after Surgery by Nicole Pecquex, MD

Bariatric Surgery continues to evolve as we search for that perfect procedure or pill that minimizes complications but produces excellent sustainable weight loss for a lifetime. Both patients and their surgeons want something that minimizes risk, pain from incisions, time out of work, and chance for failure. We have seen evolution over time from surgeries like vertical banded gastroplasty to gastric bypass to band and now to sleeve. However, we still struggle with weight regain. This has resulted in morbid obesity being recognized as the chronic disease it truly is. We now counsel new patients, quoting statistics about their one-year weight loss projections. We also focus on the possibility of weight regain, while showing them that we are still there for them should this occur. Thinking has changed from "all we have is surgery in isolation", to "we need to treat this disease with all the tools at our disposal to achieve the best weight loss". This can include medication, behavioral therapy, and exercise programs.

It is difficult for a patient to regularly visit their surgeon after weight regain when they feel they have been unsuccessful. They often feel that they have let the surgeon, program, and themselves down. We now praise those who come back seeking help, as we know this is a disease that we are partnering with them to fight. We encourage, motivate, and simply embrace them in their time of need.

Frustration is not simply relegated to the patient. It is difficult as a surgeon to see a patient come back with inadequate weight loss or weight regain. We wonder why it has happened, we investigate the surgeries performed for technical issues, and we assess whether the patient is following a healthy diet and if they are exercising. If there is a technical problem, we fix it with revisional surgery. If it's not a technical problem, often patients are converted to a different surgery or are sent for intensive medical and exercise therapy. But it is difficult for the patient to regain weight and feel they have lost control. The answer to what the best thing to do for patients who come back with this challenging problem is debated. What we see emerging is the care of the total bariatric patient. Knowing that they need sometimes all these therapies together to achieve significant body mass index (BMI) change. Bariatric and metabolic surgery will continue to evolve until we have developed a way to provide these patients with sustainable weight loss.

Nicole Pecquex, MD, FACS, FASMBS
Director Steward Centers for Weight Control
Steward St. Elizabeth's Medical Center

A Bariatric Surgeon's Perspective of Weight Regain after Surgery by William Richardson, MD

Bariatric surgery is the most effective treatment we have for obesity and most patients will have success. However, like any disease treatment there are failures. Several patterns of failure have been described and early intervention seems to be the key to successful treatment. Typically, patients have quick weight loss over the first year or so after surgery and then regain a little. I like to consider this a new weight set point. After that, the patient regains weight at different rates. Under the best circumstances, the patient will be at the normal rate of the general population. At other times, their weight regain may be abnormally fast until a new set point is reached. That new point may be considered a failure of the operation.

Although there can be anatomic causes for weight regain, it is more likely that the procedure has failed the patient, rather than that there is an anatomic complication. I say that because rates of weight loss have not been associated with bougie size during sleeve gastrectomy, and re-sleeving a sleeve has only led to moderate amounts of weight loss, at best. So, size of the stomach is not directly related to weight loss, particularly in the long term. After bypass procedures to decrease pouch size, stoma between pouch and small bowel and increasing roux limb length have led to less success than the primary procedure, so these anatomic changes are not the main cause of weight regain. The idea that patients have stretched their pouch by overeating is not likely to be the main problem with the procedure, although surgical modifications are helpful and appropriate for some patients.

The most important factor for weight regain is behavioral issues, and these can be very complex. Poor food choices can be the result of depression, loneliness, anxiety, food addiction, and emotional eating. Outside of psychological issues, patients can lose their mindfulness and start grazing, binging, or increasing liquid calorie intake. Exercise habits may be hard to initiate or maintain. Cost of quality food and gym membership/personal trainers may complicate weight stabilization. Time management for proper nutrition and exercise is a problem for all of us.

Weight regain after bariatric surgery is a very complex issue. Solutions require identifying the main causes of a patient's weight regain which is tantamount to treatment.

William S. Richardson, MD, FACS, FAMBS
Professor, University of Queensland
Section Head General Surgery, Ochsner Clinic, New Orleans, LA

Introduction

"Learn from the past and let it go. Live in today."
- Louise L. Hay

Most of my clients come to me, frustrated, confused, and dejected that the weight loss they previously had control over is gone. My goal is to ultimately help you reach your goals, learning lasting habits that you carry with you after you reach your potential. Your skills will be developed and your performance will be monitored as you advance in your journey.

- This book will help you navigate through the challenges while educating you to make better choices, toward a sustainable, and less frustrating journey.
- This book will pay attention to you and your personal goals whether it be losing weight, building muscle, increasing energy, sleeping better, or eating around restrictions.
- This book will offer you support that is crucial for your success where you never feel you are alone and have fun along the way
- This book will offer you lasting results and lifestyle changes with permanent results, building a sustainable relationship with food

Set Point Theory

With regards to obesity, there are many theories and reasons why it occurs. Many factors that are involved, such as environment, genetics, psychology, and even metabolic factors. Truly, there are many variables that will lead to obesity. It is not a one factor fits all theory after all.

One theory that explains why people tend to be overweight is called the *Set Point Theory*. According to this theory, the body has a complex system of hormones. Even more, it also has a complex system of bodily signals. These signals can control appetite, metabolism, and even digestion. Based on the theory, this complex system keeps our bodies at a steady weight or what is referred to as *set point*. Thus, when an individual reduces their food intake, the body then defends the established set point.

1

It is a physical way to cope with a period where food is less available. Some evidence supporting set point theory is:

- Ghrelin seems higher in patients who have lost weight, causing increased hunger
- Metabolic rate decreases with weight loss
- Exercise needs increase from 150 to 250 minutes per day in patients who plan to lose more weight and maintain it
- It is a struggle to keep the weight off after getting off a diet. (Farias et al.2011,85-89).

Given how diverse we are, each of us has a different set point. Our bodies have almost similar ways to manage this set point, controlling cholesterol, blood sugar, and even blood pressure. This set point is still dictated by everyone's genetic, psychological, and environmental factors. Should there be changes in any of these factors, it will lead to a higher set point that in turn can lead to more body fat storage (Farias et al.2011,85-89).

This theory also explains why diet and exercise are not enough for someone to lose weight. It is no wonder why then no matter how hard we eat less and exercise more often, reaching our desired weight can still be a difficult journey. This is because when we go on a diet, our body thinks it is being starved. When that happens, survival kicks in. This results in our body storing energy-rich body fat, hence, we don't lose weight that easily (Farias et al.2011,85-89).

But there's a way to be able to effectively lose weight. Bariatric surgery can truly make a difference. It helps to reset the body's ability to manage weight, altering its complex relationships with behavior and metabolism. This paves the way to lasting change by changing the anatomy of the stomach and the intestines which in turn can help lower appetite and keep a person satiated. Even more, this can even bypass the body's set point. (Al-Najim et al.2018,1113-14).

Inside this book, you will find

- Real patient scenarios and how they have kept the weight off after bariatric surgery
- "Lose-Your-Regain" activities to work on
- Easy to follow road maps for everybody, exactly what successful patients use
- Weight maintenance strategies so you never worry about weight regain again
- Tools to keep you focused during your weight-regain-loss journey
- All your concerns and questions answered
- Tricks and hacks on snacking smart, overcoming cravings, reducing stress levels, and staying hydrated

You and I are on this journey together as we revolutionize your weight loss after bariatric surgery. You have access to my resources and can benefit from my clinical knowledge. Welcome to the **"Weight-Regain-Losers-Club"** after bariatric surgery."

Figure One

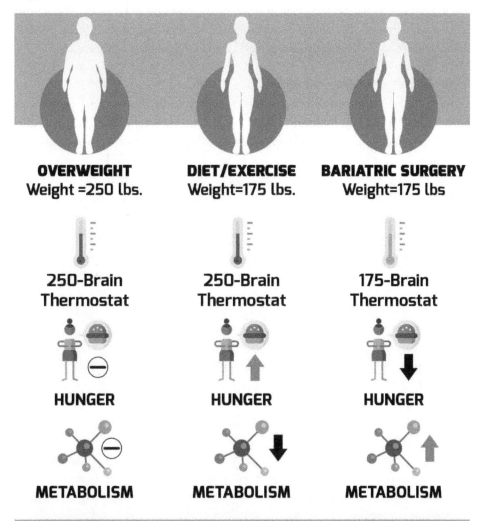

OVERWEIGHT
Weight =250 lbs.

DIET/EXERCISE
Weight=175 lbs.

BARIATRIC SURGERY
Weight=175 lbs

250-Brain Thermostat

250-Brain Thermostat

175-Brain Thermostat

HUNGER

HUNGER

HUNGER

METABOLISM

METABOLISM

METABOLISM

When the brain is most comfortable with the body, the point is known as the brain thermostat. The brain adjusts the hunger hormones and metabolism to maintain the weight at 250 lbs.

Despite diet and exercise without bariatric surgery, losing weight to 175 lbs. causes the brain to still see you as 250 lbs. leading to increased hunger and reduced metabolism. Result being, returning to the overweight stage.

The brains thermostat gets reset after bariatric surgery. This means the brain perceives you as a 175 lbs. person with hunger and metabolism staying at 175 lbs.

For many patients, shedding the pounds soon after bariatric surgery is the easy part. It's keeping it off that can be the ultimate challenge. Patients feel themselves bouncing on a trampoline, where the harder they try, the faster the weight returns. This kind of weight cycling is a common occurrence as patients progress over the years after bariatric surgery.

Pinpointing and tackling the precise reasons behind the weight regain can reverse the damage. This book reveals the most common weight maintenance saboteurs experienced by real life patients, and how they fight back against each.

The Honeymoon Period

The honeymoon period after bariatric surgery is the most crucial period you have in developing and building a bridge over troubled waters. Weight loss is dramatic during this period which may last anywhere from twelve to twenty-four months.

In the beginning, you might not understand when the bariatric team keeps emphasizing that "surgery is only a tool." The tool will continue to work till you keep working it. It may not remain as shiny and new as it once was. The manual might be a little worn out and may need additional love and care to keep it in top form. Though surgery does cause lifestyle changes to a certain extent, it still does not prevent you from eating even when you are not hungry after the honeymoon period ends (Al-Najim, et al,2018,1113-14).

If you have passed the honeymoon period and have still not figured out the reasons for your pre-operative eating habits, you have a greater chance of regaining your weight back. You risk gaining momentum with detrimental behaviors like grazing, picking, and nibbling throughout the day. "Slider food syndrome," involving processed carbohydrates like pretzels, potato chips, and crackers (foods that slide right through your pouch), gains momentum.

Figure Two

Staying on track in a culture loaded with food opportunities is not easy. Ups and downs are bound to happen and ongoing commitment is needed. It is common for patients to regain 10% to 15% of their initial excess weight loss after weight loss surgery.

However, if you regain more than this, it might be a red flag that you have not changed your lifestyle habits, are unable to manage the stress, and have given in to environmental challenges. This book might be exactly what you have been looking for.

In this book, you will learn actionable strategies that will mesh with your lifestyle to achieve lasting changes. Just eating less and exercising more is not enough.

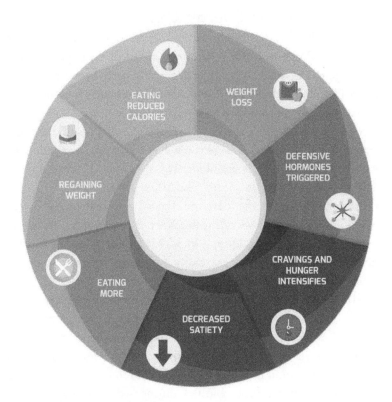

Factors like genetics, environmental cues, emotional state, and drug interactions all contribute to a person's weight regain.

Some of the challenges bariatric patients face as they move forward are:

1. <u>Weight loss stall</u>: As you lose weight after bariatric surgery, you also lower the number of calories your body needs. The key to losing more weight is to adjust your food intake and exercise regime in new ways. Prepare for inevitable plateaus by tracking your diet and activity every day.

2. <u>Expect less support</u>: When you start losing weight during the honeymoon period you are bombarded with praise and compliments. As time goes on, your weight loss is not news anymore, and the cheering squad disappears. This can lead to a lack of enthusiasm and interfere with progress. Continue to share small goals and keep inviting friends and family to celebrate your progress. Also, become your own source of rewards.

3. <u>Stressful events</u>: Bad days' lead to bad weeks which in turn lead to bad months, and before you realize it, your life is turned upside-down. Negative emotions and stress cause you to skip workouts, give in to cravings, and find yourself moving toward your pre-surgical weight. It is imperative to maintain a daily relaxation habit, to reach out for help, and to make support groups an important part of your life.

Make Peace with the Energy Gap

As you keep losing weight after bariatric surgery, even though your body does not need as many calories as it did before you started plateauing, something frustrating starts happening. Your body can't tell the difference between eating less and being stuck in a famine. Your metabolism slows and your body goes into a protective mode, stimulating your appetite to preserve fat stores.

"Energy gap" is a term that was coined to describe estimating the change in your energy balance point. This is knowledge you will need for reaching and maintaining successful body weight goals. It is useful for: 1) Prevention of excessive weight gain, and 2) Maintenance of weight loss (Hill, et al.2009, 1848-53).

- Once you lose weight after bariatric surgery, your body needs fewer calories to maintain the weight loss. This is called the "energy gap." To avoid weight-regain, the energy gap is around hundred calories or less a day. Inability to keep that energy gap going inevitably leads to the weight creeping back on. (Hill et al,2009,1848-53).
- Re-determine how many calories you consume as you lose weight. The body needs fewer calories to maintain itself as your weight goes down, and keeping track of the energy gap helps maintain weight loss.
- Avoid compensating for your workouts. Refrain from resting more than you normally would or eating higher caloric foods after working out
- Calculate the net calories burned during workouts by subtracting the number of calories you burn when not exercising. To get an accurate number of net calories burned, if during a thirty-minute workout you burned 300 calories, you would subtract the calories spent if you had been sitting (twenty -forty calories). (Hill et al,2009,1848 -53).

***

Lose-Your-Regain Activity # one: Motivate Yourself with a Mantra

Mantras can comfort and support you during your transformation, helping you achieve your goals.

An inspirational mantra is a thought that you can repeatedly say to yourself three times a day for seven days keeping you motivated and focused on a weight loss challenge. Here's how to create one:

- Think of one of your weight loss goals
- Come up with an inspirational phase or simple statement that motivates you
- Repeat it aloud when you feel discouraged, or stressed

Some ideas for motivational mantras are:

"If we don't change, we don't grow. If we don't grow, we are not really living." – Gail Sheehy

"Transformation literally means going beyond your form." – Wayne Dyer

"Motivation is what gets you started. Habit is what gets you going." – Jim Ryan

"The way you think, the way you behave, the way you eat, can influence your life by thirty to fifty years." – Deepak Chopra

"No Masterpiece was ever created by a lazy artist." – success.com

"One year equals 365 possibilities" – success.com

"The best way to get something done is to begin." – success.com

"Nothing changes if nothing changes" – Gloria Sanderson

https://go.omadahealth.com/.

(Health, Omada."The Omada Program".n.d.)

***

Now, meet Jamal, who changed his life and his health with surgery. He believed in the improbable and made it happen. He is an extraordinary example of how change rewards you when you work for it. Read about how he visualized where he wanted to be and moved toward it. It is amazing how a world can open with the thought, "I just want to live."

Figure Three

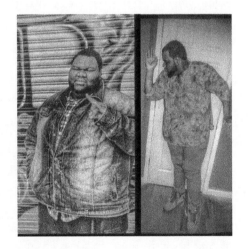

Jamal: My name is Jamal and my journey, just like everyone else, has been filled with ups and downs. But what makes my journey worth it is the fact that I have successfully added years to my life by using my surgery as a tool to help me improve. I started my journey at 586 pounds.

I stand today at 332 pounds and I'm still working toward my goals because when it comes to being healthy, everything is always under construction. There are many ways one could stay on track during their process, but what kept me going was the idea that I would have a future.

For so long, all I imagined for my future was being a grim, depressed person who was unhealthy and hated his appearance. But now, I believe that I gave myself a chance to grow old and experience life beyond food and comfort.

I get a chance at having a family and that is another thing that keeps me on track. Now, my motivation stems from the desire to be able to play with my children and help them with sports. I grew up playing sports and I feel that my future children deserve a father who will participate in their lives fully and not from the confines of a couch.

Good health is another huge motivator that keeps me on track. It's a simple idea but you'd be surprised how we lose sight of how important health is when we're thinking about food all the time. Being generally healthy is a big reason I keep going and I just want to live. I think what keeps me from going back to my old ways is the thought of an early death. I'm not afraid to die, not at all, but what I am afraid of is dying knowing I have so much to offer the world and that my death could've been prevented by simply eating healthier and exercising.

I have control and so do all of you by reading this book. During my workouts, I find it best to pace myself and not to over exert because when you over exert you become discouraged not necessarily because you can't do something but because you may be physically tired. During this journey, you will feel discouraged at points because I did myself, but you must understand that it's a battle of life and death.

I am a believer that slow and steady wins the race. I approach exercise in the same way I would approach my old eating habits. I ask myself how would I eat a Big Mac? And the answer is relatively universal, you eat it one bite at a time. That is exactly how I treat my exercise every day. Every set is one at a time, I try not to stress as much as I can since we can only control our future, never the past, so let's keep one foot in-front of the other and continue to elevate.

Setting small goals that lead to a bigger one is a good way to approach weight loss. I look at it like this – it took me several years to gain so it will take several years to lose but with hard work and dedication, I will be able to overcome the obstacles and achieve great results.

Finally, the most important piece to this puzzle will be food itself. I have learned to eat to live and not live to eat. I practice portion control because good portion control coupled with better decision making makes everything easier.

This journey is quite like building a car you must put all the pieces together carefully and precisely. Once you do that, you add gas and that will determine performance. If you put bad gas in your dream car, it won't sound or run as good. Think of your body the same way. Feed your body good things and it will be good to you. Your body is your temple so treat it as such. We've all been given the gift of life and if you have the power to save your life through better decisions, then it's important for you to do so.

Chapter One

My Story

"Pay the farmer or pay the hospital."
– Birke Baehr

I love people
   I love helping and guiding people after bariatric surgery.
   I love health and fitness and all the intricacies of weight loss.
   I guide. I coax. I motivate. I support. I talk to clients. I build dreams. I am your partner in your weight loss journey.

As a physician's assistant and registered dietitian in the field of bariatrics, I have helped an endless number of patients lose the weight that they have regained years after bariatric surgery.

I have been in the field of bariatrics since 1998, and have worked with amazing bariatric surgeons. I have never given up on my clients.

Besides being an author, my bachelor's degree is in nutrition, and I later did graduate studies to become a physician's assistant and received a master's in health care management.

When I am not working, you can usually find me out hiking the local trails, haunting the local bookstore, or exploring healthy new food products for my clients to try.

I currently live with my husband in New York, a city that provides me with constant inspiration, where I work as a bariatric coordinator.

I'm No Expert

Well, I am kind of an expert helping clients deal with weight regain after bariatric surgery. I have a bunch of letters after my name, though my most important qualification for writing this book is that I have been a part of the post-operative journey of many bariatric clients who have regained, helping them get over the speed bumps, rooting for them, and using my knowledge to approach their problems sensibly. I have tried to put everything that I believe would be helpful into this book.

When I was in school, my aunt was diagnosed with breast cancer and passed away six months later. I was extremely close to her and the shock and heartbreak made me wonder if there was anything she/we could have done to prevent or reverse the progression of the disease. In addition to obesity, diabetes and hypertension, being rampant in my family, this was something new. Though I did not jump into picking nutrition as my career path right away, it did spark a deep interest in me.

Fast forward five years later when, as a graduate student, I had a college roommate suffer a stroke at the age of twenty nine. A hectic lifestyle along with endless hours of studying, examination stress, eating from the vending machine, and having a sedentary lifestyle all led to her in the emergency room. Scans and an MRI confirmed the diagnosis.

This scary and life changing event made me decide that I wanted to help and teach people how to eat right and lead healthier lifestyles. It fueled my desire to empower and encourage my clients to put their health and wellness first. I became a registered dietitian specializing in weight loss. My physician assistant's degree was a perfect complement to probing the clinical aspects of disease in the human body.

As I became a more experienced dietitian in the field of obesity, my interest expanded to the area of bariatrics because I saw the positive impact that nutritional therapy had on patients after bariatric surgery. Unlike a one-time consultation with a dietitian, bariatric patients need ongoing, personalized support and education as they advance through the various stages of their weight loss journey.

As I sat down to write this book on weight regain after bariatric surgery, I took a lot of time to reflect on my last twenty years of clinical practice. In addition to acknowledging the good and the bad, my clients' successes and failures, I'm also reflecting on the ordinary and extraordinary. I thought about the post-operative clients who have seen me, and what they have endured during their weight loss journeys. Most of them reach out after they have suffered weight regain after bariatric surgery. Most of them are upset with themselves. Many have spent lots of time, effort and money trying to get back on track. Yet here they are, sitting across from me either in person or virtually, telling me that they are ready to do anything, give up everything to get back to their goal weight that keeps eluding them.

They are looking at me to boost their hopes and give them the necessary courage to lose the weight and lose it for good.

Life does get in the way of maintaining weight after bariatric surgery. It is just not easy, and I don't believe that you are at fault when you are in the position of struggling to lose the weight you have regained back.

I thrive on teaching and encouraging weight loss surgery patients to make healthier choices. Each day is filled with amazing teaching moments- from seeing clients learn to add more protein on their plates to having them demonstrate how to read food labels. These are the moments why I became a bariatric dietitian.

Welcome to My World

I am your guide now as I take you under my wing and lead you on this journey of punching weight regain in the face after bariatric surgery.

I will show you easy skills and strategies that you can adopt every day. Everything is easier when there are clear instructions and unlimited support, and that is exactly what you will get from me. Keep moving forward with no complicated rituals or time-consuming tasks. Watch it work for you!

Soon you will overcome past historical set points, jump start the weight loss, and keep it off altogether. I wanted to write a book that was simple to follow that will make your post- bariatric life easier. This book is the best of everything I have learned: a collection of ideas used by successful bariatric clients, ideas that will work for everyone all the time.

Be aware that there is power in you to lose weight and keep it off for life. By the end of this book you will have the necessary tools needed to prevent weight regain after bariatric surgery and have a steady weight maintenance that is doable.

I am passionate about helping people lose weight after bariatric surgery. There is no better feeling than seeing the positive changes in some one's life and celebrating those accomplishments together. Whether their goals are to get pregnant after bariatric surgery, whether it's crossing their legs when siting down, fitting into the chairs at Yankee stadium, getting off their medications, running marathons, being able to travel the world, becoming fitness instructors, playing with their kids, in short, gaining their lives back, I find nothing more rewarding or gratifying than transforming and enriching lives. I intend to have a positive, and hopefully an extraordinary impact on the lives of all my clients. I am your on-call dietitian.

Stay awesome!

Figure Four

Thinking of having surgery

Starting preoperative process

Completion of preoperative testing

Day of surgery

Honeymoon period

Weight loss goals reached

Return of old habits

Weight Regain begins

5-10 pound regain

20 pound regain

Completely off track

Giving up

Looking to have revisional surgery or looking for help

(Branao, et al.2015,122-128)

Chapter Two

Twelve Core Pillars for Losing Your Weight Regain

"To hold, you must first open your hand. Let go."
— Lao Tzu

The twelve "Weight Regain" Core Pillars

W: Will power
E: Environmental cues
I: Increase metabolism
G: Grazing, picking, and nibbling
H: Hydration
T: Tracking food intake

R: Retrain your fat cells
E: Exercising consistently
G: Glucose/insulin tolerance
A: Acceptance of portion control
I: Interactive weight loss tools
N: Never look back

I n **Chapter four,** you will understand how to tame the hunger monster with will power and delay acting upon cravings, which will weaken the strength of your cravings over time.

In Chapter five, you will explore the environmental cues surrounding you. Discover how to tackle them to help comply with your new lifestyle, and you will learn how to differentiate between social hunger, emotional hunger, and habitual hunger.

In Chapter six, you will discover the key to firing up your metabolism that has been revving at less than half the speed after your "honeymoon period" has passed.

In Chapter seven, you will adopt strategies to: stop grazing, picking, nibbling, and sabotaging yourself; gain the right mindset in snacking, and learn how to use emotional techniques to stay motivated through the ups and downs of your bariatric journey.

In Chapter eight, you will discover the importance of hydration, and understand how fluids will help you to increase energy levels and function optimally as you lose.

In Chapter nine, you will learn painless methods of looking at what you eat as part of your daily schedule, along with discovering how critical self-monitoring is for success, and increase your self-awareness of target behaviors and outcomes.

In Chapter ten, you will retrain your fat cells by releasing fat that you can use for fuel and to burn additional fat even when at rest. You will learn how to eat good fats to burn additional fat and flip the switch from fat storing to fat burning.

In Chapter eleven, you will understand that consistent exercising is crucial for successful weight loss and avoidance of weight regain. You will learn to keep your Monday commitment strong, on line and in focus all week long.

In Chapter twelve, you will learn that since insulin only burns carbohydrates, when you crave carbs you begin a vicious cycle.

In Chapter thirteen, you will learn portion control, learn how to trust your taste buds, and know that an unfinished plate is a sign that the right amount of food has been eaten.

In Chapter fourteen you will learn how to stay engaged when motivation lags, continue your healthy behavior, and discover that participating with technology is instrumental in your successful weight loss.

In Chapter fifteen, you will learn to make weight regain a distant memory by using failure to your advantage, also to recognize that a mistake is a one-time thing that can be overcome by admitting it, and to then move forward with your program.

Weight loss surgery is an awesome tool that helps you lose weight significantly, but it does not guarantee immunity to weight regain and weight loss plateaus. Your body is incredibly adaptive and does its best to maintain equilibrium. Weight loss plateaus are the biggest motivation killer and happen to most post-operative patients.

When you are fast approaching your weight loss goals, you have been going to the gym or exercising for months. You are also watching what you eat. You are happy with the previous month's results. You are seeing the scale going down whenever you weigh yourself. But, alas, today it seems that nothing is happening. One moment you're losing weight, and then suddenly the scales refuses to budge. You are doing the same thing: same amount of food, same menu, same exercise routine but still you're stuck.

You might think that doing the same thing will be beneficial to you. After all, why fix something that's working right? Well, wrong! The human body is a wonderful organism that is very adaptive to any calorie deficit. This means that it already got used to your routine, which makes it somehow complacent. Hello plateau!

The scenario stated above is really nothing new. As a matter of fact, many tend to experience a weight loss plateau. During this time, many will feel so disappointed with their weight loss journey that they will no longer commit to behavioral change, and go back to their old ways. Alas, the weight that they have shed off will eventually come back.

Yet, don't let this discourage you. If you are experiencing the same thing, there are ways to escape it. So, what should you do to skip over this frustrating period? Let me tell you the story of my client Gemma who successfully overcame a weight-loss plateau.

Gemma is one of my most committed clients. Being in her mid-twenties, she knew that her decision to undergo weight loss surgery would change the course of her life. Gemma usually makes her meals during the weekend and prepacks them in containers. It becomes more convenient for her to cook once or twice a week, so she will not be tempted to eat food from the outside. She also goes to the same indoor spin class in her gym on the way home.

However, cooking only once a week also has its downsides. She tended to use the same ingredients and would only eat two or three variations of her meal. So, after a steady weight loss, her plateau made her frustrated and she asked me for advice.

What I told her was to try the following things: food mix-up, calorie cycling, and exercise variation.

Food mix-up is somewhat self-explanatory. I advised Gemma to add a different variety of food in her diet. Instead of always eating oats for example, why not eat lentils or quinoa? Instead of snacking on fruit, try nuts as an alternative. Keep the body guessing by eating a variety of healthy options.

Calorie cycling is another great way to kick start weight loss again. What I asked Gemma to do is cycle the week into high calorie and low-calorie days. Alternating between these days can keep her metabolism working at its hardest.

A calorie cycling week would look something like this:

Figure Five

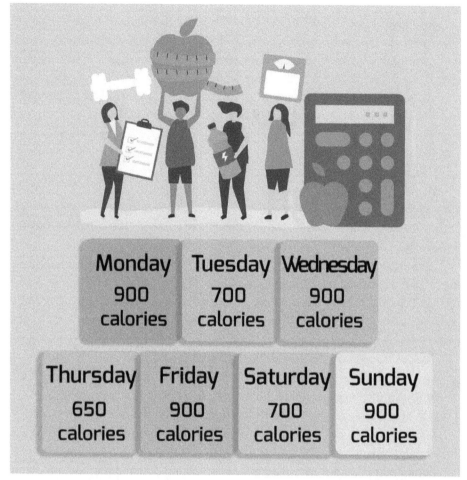

Monday	Tuesday	Wednesday
900 calories	700 calories	900 calories

Thursday	Friday	Saturday	Sunday
650 calories	900 calories	700 calories	900 calories

Also, be watchful of the amount you're eating because although you may think you're eating the same amount, you may be eating more than before. After bariatric surgery, patient appetites tend to increase with time and tend to follow the path below.

One month: Three to four bites

Six months: Three to four ounces at every meal

One year: Five to six ounces at every meal

Three years: Six to eight ounces at every meal

Five+ years: Eight to ten ounces at every meal

Exercise variation is actually very important. What I asked Gemma to do was to try other exercises available in her gym, like doing strength training exercises or maybe something fun like Zumba or a high intensity interval training (HIIT) class.

When I introduced these concepts to Gemma, she was of course a bit reluctant. I could understand this because she had already gotten into a routine and it was difficult to steer away from what had been working. But after a few weeks, Gemma was brimming with happiness, saying she was back on her weight loss journey.

***

Figure Six

START PLAYING THE ROLE OF A COACH FOR YOURSELF BY ANSWERING THE FOLLOWING QUESTIONS
with this weight regain checklist

Food:
- Are you still engaged with your dietitian?
- Are you watching your portion sizes?
- Are you taking longer than 20 minutes to eat a meal?
- What if any, carbohydrates are you not inclined to give up?
- Are you drinking your calories?
- Are you relying on slider foods and liquid meals?
- Are you grazing?
- Are you timing your meals?
- Are you eating enough protein?

Activity:
- What physical activity do you enjoy the most?
- Do you change your exercise routine periodically?
- Does exercising solo work for you or do you need accountability?
- What are your barriers to physical activity?

Schedule:
- What have you compromised on to accommodate your post-bariatric life?
- Can you delegate or recruit help to better manage your schedule?

Environment:
- Do you have cues set up to help you stay on track?
- What happens when these cues are not in place?

Motivation:
- Do you work with an effective motivating force?
- What is your support system for motivation and encouragement?

Mindset:
- Are you eating to manage emotional challenges?
- Are you able to reframe negative thoughts?
- What strategies shift your mindset and help you focus on

As your own coach, you will be able to focus on things you do well and identify things you need to change or improve by returning to these questions on a regular basis

Bringing about a change is not about trying to fight yourself, but getting so strategic that you end up winning even before the fight begins. You need to work on changing the brain before changing your body or the changes will not last.

Our bodies are a result of our brain state. After bariatric surgery, our subconscious brain drives most of our behaviors along with influencing our decisions. The way our brain changes is not easily noticeable since the change is very gradual (Jumbe et al,2015,225-42).

Attempts at change needs to start before bariatric surgery to have more success. When patients fail in attempting change, healthcare professionals look at it as laziness or a patient's lack of motivation. When, in fact, the change has not been designed according to how the brain processes change. Follow the plan by:

- Jumpstarting your metabolism
- Burning fat more efficiently
- Reducing your stress hormones
- Stabilizing insulin and blood sugar levels
- Increasing exercise
- Combating grazing and cravings

After developing the power within yourself to follow this plan, you will feel like you have flown across the country to see me at my office without ever having to leave home.

***

Lose-Your-Regain Activity # two: Better Rewards

When there is, a reward waiting for you at the end it is easier to finish a small or large task easily. Losing your regained weight is its own reward, but the little steps you take to get there along with the small goals you accomplish on the way also need to be rewarded.

Traditional rewards usually entail food and promote unhealthy eating. It does not make sense to give up soda and then reward yourself with a bowl of ice cream. Developing a new reward skill will help you pick nonfood rewards for every goal you reach on your weight loss journey.

- Brainstorm nonfood rewards on paper or on your computer/phone
- Organize the list of rewards from small to big
- Pair one of the rewards with a goal you are working toward

https://go.omadahealth.com

(Health, Omada."The Omada Program".n.d.)

Figure Seven

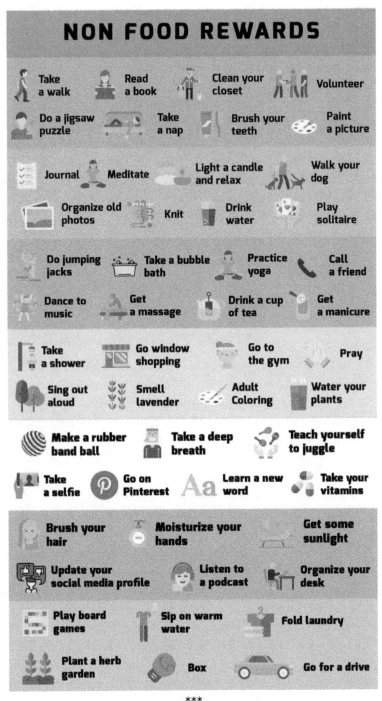

***

Meet Raquel, who had the lap band initially and found that it did not work for her as well as she would have liked. She considered revisional gastric sleeve surgery and has never looked back. Read about how she creates a habit of success for herself and builds her list of accomplishments to stay in a positive frame of mind. Prove to yourself, you get done what you make up your mind to do.

Figure Eight

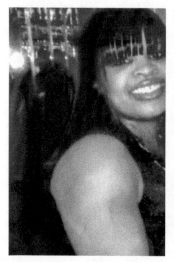 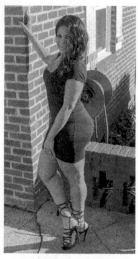

Raquel: Sometimes it's tough when you're asked to put your weight loss journey in words because the emotions involved are more prevalent than one could ever explain. Being overweight, having my body mass index (BMI) classify me as obese or severely obese has been my world since I was a child. It is something I struggled with all my life since I could remember.

I always really wanted to be this beautiful, slim, pretty girl. My mother was a model, tall, and beautiful and my dad was a tall, slim, and handsome man. I could never figure it out, but always questioned, "Wait, how did I miss that gene?!"

I felt cheated, ugly, and just angry at the way I looked. As I got older, combating this weight issue became more and more important. As I became an adult, and financially self-sufficient, I poured so much money into losing weight. I did all the fad diets, took prescription diet pills, over the counter diet pills, and any other diets that were available at the time. Yup, they all worked, but all these things were just temporary.

In 2002, I met the man of my dreams. I was overweight, but he accepted me for who I was. In 2004, he proposed, I accepted and next thing you know, this fat girl was planning her wedding. So, of course, in my head, I was not going to walk down the aisle a fat girl and have these fat girl pictures to reference for the rest of my life. I envisioned myself in the sexiest wedding dress ever.

So, I found my dress before I lost the weight and ordered it in the size I wanted to be. The store made me sign for this as they though it was a drastic move. Who does this? But in my head, I know how to lose weight and had done this before. "I got this." So, I signed it. When it was time to pick up my dress, they were all amazed as I could fit in this dress, and with no corset! Again, like all other weight loss attempts and success, I was happy and so proud of myself.

As time went on, I went back to my old eating ways and gained all the weight I lost back, plus a few extra pounds. So back on the diet I went. However, during this time with the weight gain also came hypertension, and then medication to control the hypertension. I was quickly approaching forty years old, and that's when I knew that I needed to do something to get my weight under control.

Weight loss surgery was always an option, but I was concerned about what people would think about me and questioned if I was big enough to get it. Although at that time I was about 218 pounds, my highest weight was about 228, and my research said I just was not heavy enough for the surgery. What I didn't know was that hypertension was considered a comorbidity and reduced the BMI required for weight loss surgery. It was at this point I said to myself, this is the answer to all my problems.

In the summer of 2008, I made my appointment to see the surgeon and decided on the lap band for weight loss. I didn't tell many people, but with my husband's blessings, I went for it. So, February 4, 2009 was the day!!

Initially I was losing weight quickly. I was very excited. Every time I went to see my surgeon, I reported to him how much I loved my lap band and then after about losing forty five pounds I hit a plateau. I became comfortable with eating whatever I wanted, just small portions. I felt like this was the purpose of the surgery and if I eat less, I would lose weight, right? Nope, wrong! What I quickly learned was that the lap band or any weight loss surgery is not a quick fix. It is a surgical tool that one must use to assist them in losing weight.

During this process, I realized that my relationship with food had to change for my life to change. This process was no longer a fad diet, but it had become a lifestyle as everything depended on it. But I was not perfect all the time! I had several relapses and with that came weight gain. I never gained back anything close to what I lost, but any amount of weight gain was too much in my eyes.

I had a lot of problems with my lap band, and due to some medical complications, I had it removed in June of 2017. It was now I had to challenge myself more than ever because gaining weight was the last thing I needed to do. I gained back approximately ten pounds, but it was better than a hundred pounds.

In October of 2017, I did a conversion to the Gastric sleeve. It has been the best thing that I have done. The sleeve is very different from the lap band, and has proven to be the right tool for me. I could get within thirteen pounds of my goal weight since I had my sleeve. I attempt to eat nutritious meals and make good decisions most of the time, I have incorporated exercise in my daily routine and attend support groups as this is not something I could do alone. I get cravings, but I don't deprive myself of them. If I want something, I eat it, but I always stay in moderation and I move on.

As my body changed, my mind changed with it. I love the way I look in clothes. I love the compliments I receive, and I am more excited that I am no longer taking medication for my high blood pressure. I now love the new me! I have many weak moments, many times I have indulged, because I am not perfect, but I am a daily work in progress!! My highest weight was 228, my surgery weight was 218, my current weight before the plastic surgery was 165, and my goal weight is 150 pounds.

I struggle daily with making good food choices cause like most people I love the taste of most things that are not good for you. However, someone once said in the support group, "Nothing tastes as good as skinny feels!" And I strongly believe that.

However, my favorite quote that keeps me focused, simply says, "The ability to discipline yourself to delay gratification in the short term to enjoy greater rewards in the long term is the indispensable prerequisite for success".

Chapter Three:
Will Power and
The Hunger Monster

Lack of direction, not lack of time, is the problem.
We all have twenty-four-hour days
–Zig Ziglar

Will power is a hard concept to understand. Looking for will power and coming up short? Many people demonstrate will power in various parts of their life but are unable to use it in losing weight. It is a combination of impulse control and motivation.

- Willpower decreases when you get inadequate sleep.
- Willpower increases when you feel good about yourself.
- Willpower decreases when you are a caretaker.
- Willpower increases when you eat something good for yourself.
- Willpower decreases when you are stressed.
- Willpower increases when you are busy, but not stressed.
- Willpower decreases when family and friends tempt you.
- Willpower increases when the weather is warm and the sun is bright.

Impulse control is that automatic feeling of reaching for a slice of pizza or ice cream as it moves toward you like a magnet and your hand is made of steel. Resisting this feeling is impulse control. Though this behavior is a little bit genetic, you can still train yourself to resist it. Will power is necessary, but unfortunately, it's often temporary. The best motivation is when you find the desire to change yourself in a more fundamental, long-lasting manner. (Leahey et al,2012,84-91).

Imagine your life without the presence of impulse control issues:

- You stay focused until you complete an entire task without getting distracted.

- Any temptation and addiction to food, alcohol, shopping, and Netflix binging disappears
- The word "procrastination" does not exist when you plan your exercise schedule

Not so easy! It is very difficult to change one's behavior, create new habits, and eliminate bad ones.

When you are trying to manage your weight loss, it's easy to perceive hunger as that monster waiting to sabotage your weight loss efforts. The hunger monster is unleashed when you skip meals and deprive yourself of food, and when you lavish it with constant snacks and increased portion sizes. Taming this beast is the best alternative, forcing it to work for you, rather than work against you.

Master your hunger and make it your friend by:

- Spotting the true signs of hunger: Learn to recognize what exactly makes your hunger monster tick. Is it stress, boredom, or just giving up?
- Taking it slow: Eating slowly and a little less than usual, will set you up for a steadier weight loss, nudging the hunger monster to the side
- Eat slow release foods: Rather than filling up with sugary and high carbohydrate foods, opt for fiber, and complex carbohydrates like quinoa or oatmeal, which keeps the hunger monster happy till the next meal
- Mistaking thirst for hunger: Always drink a glass of water twenty to thirty minutes before you eat.
- Watch the snacks: Throwing snacks at the hunger monster will cause a blow out, increase hunger and the desire to eat.
- **Let go of fear: Do not let the hunger monster scare you. Start feeling more comfortable with hunger pangs. Don't feel like you must satisfy them right away. Gain control over it.** (Leahey et al,2012,84-91).

Willpower Alone Is Not Enough for Weight Loss

You consciously act by the help of two mechanisms: **motivation and willpower**. While motivation is the desire to act, willpower is the desire to act regardless of how one feels.

When you lose weight after bariatric surgery, biological factors come into play, making it difficult for you to keep the weight loss off after it has gone. Being successful or unsuccessful at keeping weight loss at bay is not a reflection of one's willpower reserve. When you lose a tremendous amount of weight after bariatric surgery, your metabolism gets out of whack, leading to an increase in appetite, where for every two pounds lost, you eat hundred calories more. (Leahey et al,2012,84-91).

What is the usual scenario with regards to food restrictions? We indeed lose some weight, but then our weight loss, plateaus. Our old weight comes back as if nothing happened. This is typical most especially in the show "The Biggest Loser." During the program the participants are losing tremendous weight. But when they are already out from the competition, they gain most of their weight back.

This is a dramatic example of how our bodies fight against weight loss. Hence, sheer willpower can barely help.

"Why is that we can't just control our body weight?" You can decide whether to take that next bite of breakfast, right? Why can't we just keep that going over years? The answer is that your brain, like several poorly run institutions, is governed by a committee."

This can be attributed to the brain's wirings with regards to its reward system. Our brain is programmed to find cake a much better reward than a carrot stick. The brain's hypothalamus is our body's weight thermostat. It prefers the body to be of a certain weight, which is referred to as the set point. The moment our weight dips or even increases, hunger and even our calories will be adjusted to bring it back to its normal state. And this is always active (Farias et al,2011,85-89).

Also, involved here is the executive system. This deals with our decision making and planning. The secret weapon for weight loss takes a lot of vacations. Studies show that willpower can be very taxing for people. It is no wonder then that it is harder for us to control our urges. This executive system will not do better whenever we are lonely and stressed. The basic answer to why people have so much trouble with losing regained weight is that they're so hung up on using a system that tires easily to fight against brain systems that are always working, never taking a day off.

What are we going to do then?

The answer can be relatively simple. Just choose healthier habits, from food to exercise. These habits will yield a healthier result, and can somehow help us reach our ideal body mass index. Eating mindfully and listening attentively to the body will help us steer clear from unhealthy food choices.

There's always a point in our life that the only thing that will push us forward would be willpower. Yet, even if we have a dose and a ton of it, it seems we too get tired. And this can have adverse effects. Whenever we feel the weight of life tugging us down, we tend to succumb to night- time cravings, such as heading to the nearest coffee shop or even eating a whole bag of chips.

Fluctuating willpower should not be a concern at all. For you to be able to sustain it with the right amount of energy, here are three foundations that can help you along the way.

1: Goal. Setting a clear goal would be a motivation for you should you tend to lose your strength and willpower. Setting an undefined goal will cause confusion and the journey to realize it might go haywire. The basics in goal setting should be SMART. This means it must be specific, measurable, achievable, realistic, and timely.

When establishing your goal, make sure that it fits the criteria stated above. Even more attach a number to it. For instance, if you aim to lose weight you need to add numbers to it. Exactly how much lost weight do you desire? What percentage should you want to get rid of? Are you aiming for a twenty-four-inch waist? Knowing these numbers will make your goal specific and measurable. But you also need to be able to realize if these numbers and percentages can indeed be achieved given your current state.

2: Commitment. When your goal has already been defined, it is now time to commit. For instance, if you desire to reach that twenty-four-inch waist, that won't happen overnight. Hence, you need to be able to research and find ways exactly how you can be able to do just that. You may want to reach out to your fitness friends or contact your local gym and ask around about what possible routines they can be able to provide to reach your goal. Commitment is a combination of accountability with a set of timelines. After all, we would want to be able to reach that goal in a matter of "x" number of weeks and months.

3: Environment. The next best thing to consider would be your environment. You must be conscious of it and understand yourself better. Your physical environment must also be programmed to help you reach your goal. For instance, your refrigerator and pantry must not be filled with non-bariatric friendly foods. Go out and shop for healthy food choices so you won't be tempted to eat those things and instead, eat healthy.

These are just three foundations to live by to guarantee success with any endeavor possible. First, know your goal. Second, make sure you fully commit to realizing the goal, and finally make your environment as an enabler to reach it.

Figure Nine

Food cravings have very little to do with hunger, and have both biological and psychological components. Willpower is a great thing to have, but it's not like you can flip a switch and have more of it when you need it. There are physiological and psychological factors that cause your willpower to rise and fall. Your willpower response is a reaction created by an internal conflict. Cravings have nothing to do with will power and have a mind of their own.

The Craving Whisperer

One minute, you are focused, busy, and innocently going about your day. The next minute everything changes, and you suddenly find yourself in the clutches of a chocolate cupcake with buttercream icing. You are done licking the frosting off your fingers and you are looking for more.

What happened? Well you just got clobbered by a food craving.

WILLPOWER CHEAT SHEET

When we are hit with food cravings, we give in easily, since our brains promise that it will be rewarding. We are left with regret, disappointment and additional cravings. Break the craving cycle by asking yourself the following questions:

1

Is giving in to this craving worth delaying my weight loss benefit?

The indulgence might be tempting but you want other things even more

2

How do I address the underlying issue?

Are you bored, lonely, stressed or seeking comfort?

3

How can you tell if this choice supports or impacts your life time goals?

State the facts and engage the logical part of your brain

5

You are in control of your craving. Observe it without resistance and it will subside.

Breathe slowly, and notice how it feels in your body.

4

How can I strengthen my ability to forgo easy decisions and opt for harder, long term ones?

Build dedication, and hard work through small daily efforts.

https://go.omadahealth.com
(Health, Omada. "The Omada Program". n.d.)

Cravings are a persuasion in our daily lives. They play a vital role in nudging us toward certain food choices that made us feel good in the past. Despite those choices not being consistent with our current weight loss journey, cravings are a state of mind that contribute to addictions and weight regain. A craving does not make us hungrier but makes us desire it specifically (Leahey. et al, 2012, 84-91).

Cortisol, the stress hormone, peeps its ugly head up when one is under pressure. This slows down the metabolism of food. Also, cravings for fat and sugar-laden foods increase when the weight loss-derailing choices kill hard-earned weight loss wins. This deadly combination of a stress-induced slower metabolic rate and high calorie cravings results in significant weight regain.

Stop the Cravings

Hydrate Yourself. When you deprive yourself of water, this can present itself as hunger. And when you are hungry, it is very easy to get that snack out from the pantry. Whenever you feel hungry, reach out for a glass of water because your body might be playing tricks on you. It might be you are just dehydrated rather than hungry.

Food Shopping. Make a checklist of healthier alternatives before you even head out to get groceries. As much as possible, do not food shop when you are hungry and even moody. This can lead to unhealthy food choices and you could easily give in to your cravings. Stick to the list when you head out to ensure you are not getting something unhealthy and unnecessary.

Healthy Stress Relievers. We often rely on snacks whenever we are stressed. Food is our little heaven amidst the chaos. Yet, the foods we choose are the ones adding inches to our waist. Instead of doing stress eating, find healthier alternatives to release it away. Plus, you'll gain points if you don't even involve food; try, for instance yoga, music, exercise or going out with friends.

Beat the Craving at Its Own Game: Cravings specifically use the part of the brain involved in sights and smells. A Study at McGill University revealed that visualizing a vivid picture like the details on a rainbow, engaged the same areas of the brain, thereby reducing cravings. Use visual imagery like your favorite pair of shoes, your dream home etc. to take your mind off the craving (Knäuper et al,2011,173-78).

Whiff stress away by sniffing essential oils like jasmine, mint or calendula to intercept the craving desire.

These strategies have proven time and again to combat cravings when they hit. Remember, this is your body that we are talking about. We are what we eat after all. (Drewnowski et al,1989,90182).

***

Food scientists are hired to create certain foods that are so delicious with just the right amount of everything that you struggle to stop yourself from overeating. Hyper-palatable foods cause cravings, overconsumption, and lack of willpower along with impulse buying. Unfortunately, these foods are high in sugar, fat, caffeine, and sodium, and low in nutrients. Many hyper-palatable foods are altered in the same manner as addictive drugs. The active ingredients from these hyper-palatable foods are more quickly absorbed in the blood stream leading to a higher level of reward. (Gearhardt et al.2011,140-145).

Stimuli Stacking

People are encouraged to eat when the food offers us flavors that are favored by our taste buds. These danger foods consist of the following flavors:

- Sugar
- Fat
- Salt

Combining two or more flavors, or even all three flavors like a salted caramel brownie creates a hyper-palatable food that is irresistible. You get:

- The COMFORT of fat and sugar found in ice cream, baked goods, and cookies
- The SATISFACTION of fat and salt found in fries, chips, and nachos
- The IRRESISTABILITY of fat, salt, and sugar in fries with ketchup, a salted caramel brownie and caramel popcorn.

The "Big five" are stimuli stacking interventions that create havoc with our taste buds. They consist of:

- Strong flavor
- Caloric density
- Effortless chewing
- Easily dissolvable
- Immediate deliciousness

High protein foods and veggies require about twenty chews per mouthful, which helps you keep track of your satiety signals and force you to listen to your hunger cues. Would you ever overeat Brussel sprouts?

On the other hand, processed foods need ten chews or less per mouthful, where the experience is over early and you keep wanting more (Avena et al,2011,367-368).

***

Lose-Your-Regain Activity # three: Walking Off a Craving

When you crave for unhealthy food, the craving passes with time, whether you like it or not. Once a craving hit's you, if you can hold off for ten to fifteen minutes, it starts fading. You can avoid unnecessary calories and the guilt that comes with it when you wait out a craving.

Waiting is not the easiest thing in the world, and you need to distract yourself for those tough few minutes. One perfect way to spend it is to go for a walk and start burning calories rather than consuming them. This will not only change the mood but also give you a flush of energy.

How to do it?

Every time you get a craving for the next five days, stop what you are doing right away and go rack up some steps.

https://go.omadahealth.com (Health, Omada."The Omada Program".n.d.)

***

Meet Frank and read about his weight loss success story. Frank makes it a point to attend almost every support group and stay engaged with the team. He believes this helps him stay on track and adopt the healthy lifestyle he chose when he decided to have gastric sleeve surgery. Read about how he does not wait to be inspired before he acts. Seldom does anything happen, if you wait for inspiration. Take small actions toward your goals, whether you want to or not.

Figure Ten

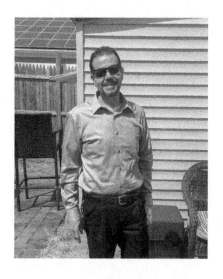

- Starting weight, 320 pounds.
- Lowest weight, post-op, 162 pounds.
- Average weight: 168-170 pounds.

Frank: I feel that my willpower is fueled by my constant desire to enjoy the benefits of the result, such as walking and having a better quality of life.

I try to keep my mission new and exciting by always making it the first and last part of my day. How? By weighing myself first thing in the morning and the last thing at night. This allows me to reflect on my day's choices. It keeps me on my best behavior. Like a first date, you are always on your game, and want to impress, but the one you are impressing is yourself! I allow myself a two to three pounds normal fluctuation, anything more puts me into a panic mode to regroup and rethink and readjust. It's easier to adjust three pounds that day, than fifteen pounds at the end of the week.

After the first year of this obsessive behavior, it becomes a way of life. You automatically eat healthy foods, you forget about the foods that you were told not to eat after surgery and they are no longer a tempting bad habit. My go-to foods and snacks are the ones that I was re-trained on.

I never test myself to see If I can handle a little of bad food because I accepted the fact that self-control and moderation with trigger foods is something that I don't have and I don't want to go back to a lifelong battle with bad habits. I obviously can't make my own rules because my history proves that, so I follow the rules that I was taught.

Support group meetings are very important to me. I attend and speak at as many as possible. This keeps the motivation new and alive. It keeps me on point and reminds me of things I forgot or take for granted. It adds to my strength and keeps me focused. Since people are very judgmental, they will be the first ones to say, "See he gained the weight back", or, "I see you're eating pasta or drinking beer, etc." So why not use human nature to your advantage?

Another benefit of meetings is that I get inspiration from my fellow bariatric friends who are losing weight and working on challenges. I also pay special attention to people that I have met who have regained weight or feel that the surgery failed them. I like to relearn from those mistakes before they happen to me.

One of the most common things that I hear is that they never gave up the bad foods. I feel that they didn't re-train their eating habits to embrace new foods and I'm sorry to say that their desire to achieve and hold on to a healthier life was not as strong or important as the desire to have that one piece of cake which could have started a downward spiral. Therefore, I try to keep it new and exciting and a priority in my life.

In summary, I believe that by thinking of it as a first date, I keep it new, keep it alive, making my weight loss the most important part of my life, because the bottom line is that it is YOUR life! And there is no end to this journey, it is only a beginning.

Chapter Four:

Environmental Cues

"Leap and the net will appear."
– John Burroughs

Most people believe that to change their environment, they need to accomplish their goals first. Comments I hear a lot are:
- If I get fitter, I could exercise more.
- If my work schedule gets better, I could meal prep.
- If I did not have such a long drive home, I would drink more water.

The main reason one is driven to eat in excess at social events and vacations is that there are too many tempting options. The brain is constantly being bombarded with cues to mimic what everyone else is doing, even if it takes a toll on the post bariatric surgery body. The "mirror effect" triggers the neurons in the brain to reflect the same emotions of people you are surrounded by (Wimmelman et al.,2014).

Environmental cues are the objects around us that trigger certain desires, thoughts, and behaviors. Environmental cues like package size, shape of plate, social presence, and lighting play a prominent role in increasing our consumption of food (Wimmelman et al.,2014).

Our environments dictate our actions. The more desirable the choices, the harder it gets to make the right decisions.

It is a misconception that change comes only from within. We overlook the fact that an optimized environment helps us make better choices and has a huge impact on our actions.

While food choice decisions determine what we eat (protein or carbohydrate), intake volume decisions determine how much we eat (three ounces or six ounces).

Brian Wansink, an expert on changing eating behavior, discusses how the size of your plate alters how much you serve yourself. While three ounces of chicken on a ten-inch plate looks like a full plate, it would look like an appetizer on a twelve-inch plate.

When do you know when to stop eating? According to Wansink, studies have indicated that a visual reminder of how much someone has eaten, tends to influence how much they eat. If chicken bones or pistachio shells are left on the table, the person remembers how much they have eaten and this influences further eating decisions. (Wansink and Sobal,2007).

***

Mindless Eating: The Future of Being Present

- Do you find yourself watching television and eating chips out of a bag?
- Do you sit at work in front of a computer and have a bowl of candy?
- Do you munch on popcorn out of a bucket at the movies, while engrossed in the movie?

Mindless eating happens when calories are consumed while the individual is unaware of the quantity that is being eaten. It adversely impacts weight loss goals and contributes to weight gain. When you base your eating decisions on emotions, it leads to frustration during your weight loss journey.

Curbing mindless eating is crucial to identifying your underlying tendencies. Focus on planning an attack to deal with stress, and brainstorm various outlets to be more productive. Pre- portioning out your servings and not arriving hungry at a social event may minimize mindless eating.

As per Dr. Brian Wansink, some strategies to help you overcome mindless eating are:

- Replacing your twelve-inch plate with a ten-inch plate: Just a two-inch plate difference leads to 22% fewer calories being consumed.
- Repackage your bigger packages into smaller Ziploc bags or Tupperware containers.
- See everything on your plate before you eat it. This causes you to eat less.
- Make visual illusions work for you, using smaller utensils, and slender glasses
- Have serving dishes placed six feet or more away from you, making it inconvenient to walk back to the kitchen for second helpings (Wansink and Sobal, 2007).

***

On the other hand, mindfulness refers to the act of being aware of your surroundings and being in the moment. Being mindful encourages you to notice any preoccupations and gently brings you back to the present. Being mindful helps you introduce moderation and restraint to your eating habits.

During your bariatric journey try to adopt mindfulness by:

1. **Sitting down** when eating your meals: Eating when driving, or on the go could cause you to choke on your meals, and lose track of how much you are eating
2. **Reflect on your feelings**: Take a moment to reflect on how you feel, and what your wants and needs are. After a moment of reflection, you can then choose to eat
3. **Chew each bite**: Take your time to enjoy the texture and flavor of foods by chewing twenty to twenty-five times a bite. This prevents you from overeating and lets you know when you are full.
4. **Cancel your membership to the Clean Plate Club**: If you are full, pack the leftovers away or just leave the last few bites. Eating beyond feeling full will cause nausea and vomiting.
5. **Switch hands**: Switching the fork from one hand to the other, slows down your eating and compels you to eat with mindfulness
6. **Critique your food**: Act like a food critic and pay attention to every little flavor and sensation of each bite

Practice mindfulness during your bariatric weight loss journey to bring greater peace and happiness into your life.

Tammy St. Clair, a clinical social worker/therapist, uses Kabat-Zinn's definition of mindfulness, to share four tools, and embarrassing stories about how she learned to do this every day. Jon Kabat-Zinn, the father of mindfulness, first wrote about mindfulness way back in 1994 (Kabat-Zinn, 1994), and has been teaching it for years before that. His definition is: "paying attention in a particular way: on purpose, in the present moment, and nonjudgmentally." (Kabat-Zinn, 1994).

Tool # one: Show up (on purpose)

Tammy first learned "to show up." It is said that 90% of success is simply showing up – and she found that to be true. She showed up every month for adjustments to her Lap-Band for nearly two years. She showed up to the support group the practice offered every month. She showed up to a therapist's office every week. She showed up to online groups where patients gathered to support one another daily. She showed up to events in Seattle while she lived in New York City. She did not underestimate the amount of support that is necessary to change her entire state of being.

Tool # two: Listen (paying attention in the present moment)

With all the showing up that Tammy did, she learned to listen – mainly to herself. She listened to her body (Was she hungry? Was she full? Why is her nose running? She was sighing, what does that mean?). She learned to listen to her mind (What's hungry, her belly, her mouth, her head?). She learned to listen to her band (too loose? Too tight?). She learned to listen to her hunger and thirst. She learned to listen to her emotions. Learning to listen is hard – there is a cacophony of noise in her brain most of the time, and she was not alone. You know you have noise too! It's uncomfortable. It challenged her assumptions. It made her heart hurt and she wanted to eat something to avoid listening. Thirteen years later, she still thinks she wants to eat when she really wants to be heard. Hear your own voice.

Listening is a key tool to long-term success.

Tool # three: Acknowledge (nonjudgmentally in the present moment)

So, the four-year-old on the inside is demanding something. Standing in the middle of the grocery store cookie aisle or freezer section (what is she doing here?), screaming at the top of her lungs and refusing to move forward unless the favorite chocolate cream-filled cookie or pint of ice cream is placed in the grocery cart and heading for immediate consumption upon paying for it.

"Ugh, what do you want now?" she frustratedly inquires as her internal four-year-old whines "but I waaaaaant it!". Having learned to listen intently to her inner child, instead of dismissing or ignoring it, Tammy has learned her language of heartaches and speedy breaths. The things that pain and annoy her or make her feel alienated or alone; even something to celebrate. Acknowledging that thought or feeling – without any "dismissal, guilt or shame" attached to it is a powerful way to show up and listen to your own needs. Acknowledging that she was hurt that she wasn't included in an invitation; acknowledging that she was angry that her boss had unattainable expectations and won't listen; acknowledging and celebrating that she lost ten pounds (the dichotomy is blinding). Once she acknowledges the thought or feeling, she is now in the position to choose how she wants to respond. This one simple act moves her from reacting in the familiar way to responding in a new way. From powerless to powerful. Acknowledging what is going on inside, in the present moment, positions her to change her behavior and to succeed. It puts her in the driver's seat and not somewhere else.

Tool # four: Get up, don't give up *(on purpose – in the present moment – non-judgmentally).*

Tammy had to accept it; she was not perfect. Darn it – she should be much better at this; since she is not and it's hard, she gives up. This is what she used to say and do when it came to her weight and losing it. "That's it, I had cake today – I might as well eat the lasagna too. I guess I'll start again on Monday." Um, what happened to the moments between now and Monday? The space/time continuum swallowed them up? She told herself "Come on, get up right now. Start again, right now." This is called resilience. And, resilience is another key to success in this journey. She learned to get up, acknowledge what caused her to trip and fall, and go again.

Tammy thinks of it often like a baby learning to walk – therefore becoming a toddler. A baby learns to roll over, sit up, crawl on all fours, and then to stand on these two little feet underneath this big body. From standing, to taking a few steps along furniture for support. A baby never learns to walk without falling – more often than they stand up sometimes – but they learn to get back up. She had to learn to nonjudgmentally acknowledge that she might have fallen but she was getting up. And kicking at whatever tripped her up in the first place! Ah, the frustration of learning through experience.

***

Mindful eating is a practice deeply rooted in Buddhist teachings which guides you to become aware of your environmental cues in satisfying your taste for food and its nourishment for the body. Eating mindfully, is essentially meditating on food and eating.

A study conducted at the Fred Hutchinson Cancer Research Center has shown a strong connection between mindful eating and practicing yoga. (Framson et al. 2009,1439-444))

Figure Eleven *(see next page)*

***

Bariatric patients have vastly differing relationships with alcohol after bariatric surgery. While some are mindfully tuned into their alcohol consumption, and enjoy alcohol mindfully and responsibly, others struggle in maintaining mindful self-awareness.

Alcohol is not recommended after bariatric surgery for various reasons. Alcohol offers empty calories and works against any weight loss goal. It is absorbed faster, causing patients to reach higher alcohol levels in the body.

The sad news is when you have an alcoholic drink you burn less fat. Studies show that a couple of martinis can reduce your fat burning ability by up to seventy percent. (Liangpunsakul et al, 2010 ,670-75)

Alcohol is a liquid carbohydrate offering seven calories/gram of alcohol. In addition to eventually leading to subsequent weight regain, alcohol interferes with absorption of water-soluble vitamins like B1(Thiamine), B6 (Pyridoxine), B12 (Cobalamin), and folate. (Liangpunsakul et al, 2010 ,670-75)

EAT LIKE A YOGI

AS PER JONNY KEST THE NATIONAL DIRECTOR OF LIFE TIMES YOGA –TEACHER TRAINING PROGRAM, THERE ARE 8 PRINCIPLES OR GUIDELINES THAT YOGIS (PEOPLE WHO PRACTICE YOGA) FOLLOW. THE WORD "YOGA" MEANS TO "YOKE' OR "TO JOIN" SYMBOLIZING AN INTIMATE RELATIONSHIP WITH ONE'S BODY.

A BARIATRIC MEAL IS VERY MUCH LIKE A YOGI MEAL WHERE CONNECTING DEEPLY WITH YOUR SENSES AND SIGNALS BRINGS INCREASED AWARENESS AND JOY IN THE LIFE OF A BARIATRIC PATIENT. EVEN IF YOU DO NOT PRACTICE YOGA, START EATING LIKE SOMEONE WHO DOES.

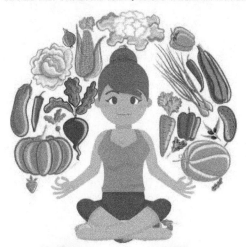

BREATHE	**STAY SEATED**	**ELIMINATE DISTRACTIONS**	**PORTION CONTROL**
Let your breath be a guide to make meal time a period of relaxation and attention.	You commit strongly to being aware of quiet time and all the subtle sensations that arise around you	Focus on the color, temperature, texture and taste of food. Free your attention from distractions to fully experience chewing your food.	Place 3 Oz of food on your plate. Finish eating it, wait a few minutes before you decide on seconds.

SLOW DOWN	**SWALLOW BEFORE YOU SPEAK**	**SAVE ROOM**	**REST AND DIGEST**
Chew your food well to give your body time to determine whether its full or not. Eating too much, too fast leads to discomfort and regret later	Pay attention to your meal and swallow first to give people at the table meaningful responses.	Leave ample room in your pouch for digestion. Eat only 80% of your pouch capacity and do not override the body	When your meal ends, be done with eating. Allow your body to digest and listen to your body.

Figure Twelve

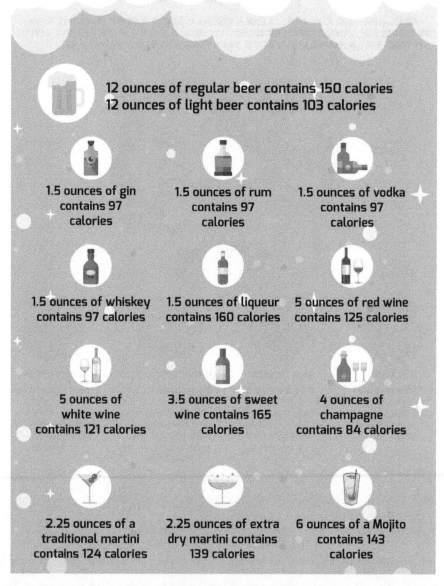

Adapted from National Institute on alcohol abuse and alcoholism .
Accessed May 03,2019.
www.rethinkingdrinking.niaaa.nih.gov/tools/calculators/calorie-calculator.aspx.

Although alcohol cravings might just come out of nowhere, they are mostly triggered by environmental situations. Negative as well as positive emotional states trigger the use of alcohol.

Mindful drinking as the name indicates is a conscious approach to consuming alcohol. (Yoder et al. 2017,717-24).

The Art of Mindful Drinking

Having personal guidelines and maintaining self-awareness is the key to having a healthy relationship with alcohol after bariatric surgery. No single guideline applies to every bariatric patient or every situation. The goal is to be able to gauge your body's response to a drink and adjust it accordingly. Your body is more sensitive to alcohol after bariatric surgery than it was before.

Carrie Wilkens, cofounder and clinical director of the Center for Motivation and Change in New York City recommends asking yourself the following questions to evaluate where you stand:

- **When do you drink?** Is it a part of every social interaction? Is it automatic or frequent?
- **Why do you drink?** Is it to cope with a stressful situation, to unwind, or to fit into your social circle of friends?
- **How easy is it to take a break?** If you are unable to stop drinking for a few days or a period, it might mean emotional or physiological dependence. (Wilkens, Carrie https://www.smartrecovery.org/tag/carrie-wilkens/.)

Wilkens, offers the following strategies in cultivating moderation:

- Taking a week off where after you set a moderation goal for each week.
- Drinking only with food to prevent a drink from going straight to your head.
- Not drinking when feeling down: Find alternative ways to deal with depression or loneliness. (Wilkens, Carrie https://www.smartrecovery.org/tag/carrie-wilkens/.)

Have you ever wondered why when you drink alcohol, there's always the presence of fatty food around you? This is because alcohol aids in making us crave calorie-rich foods. These food choices are burgers, pizza, chips, and more. Alcohol can also boost our appetite, making us want to consume more food in the process. For every drink, you must be ready to subtract calories from your meals or log another mile on the treadmill, otherwise risk weight gain.

Strategies for Scaling Back

When drinking starts feeling more urgent than relaxing after bariatric surgery, check out these tools which researchers have found to be helpful in shifting the focus away from alcohol and toward healthier behaviors.

Moderation Management
1. Make a list of problems drinking has caused
2. List of benefits you hope to gain with moderate drinking
3. Identify and manage triggers that lead to overdrinking
4. Launch new activities that can fill the drinking time

Harm Reduction
1. Name your objectives like drinking more safely, and reducing drinking
2. Come up with a plan to get there
3. Keep a log of how much you drink
4. Hydrate frequently to lower your blood alcohol content
5. Add abstinence days to your week.
6. Set time limits like starting later and ending earlier

(Wilkens, Carrie https://www.smartrecovery.org/tag/carrie-wilkens/.)

***

Vacations bring up images of exotic cocktails, extravagant buffets, and decadent desserts, but for the post bariatric patients these are not the best options. You want to stay on target with your goals and this involves a lot of planning. Just because you are on vacation, it does not mean your weight loss guidelines must be too.

How to Keep Track of What You Eat During Vacation

When you're in a foreign place, it's hard to keep track of what you eat. Planning is crucial especially with strict guidelines when travelling. On top of that, people rarely plan to stick to food protocols when they go on vacation.

- The number one rule to follow if you want to keep track of what you want to eat is to avoid the local fast food chains that offer burgers, fries, and hotdogs
- Stick with high protein, low carb snacks. Stash a few snacks in your carry on. Road trippers can stock a cooler or insulated lunch bag for the road.
- Don't forget to hydrate
- Pack your vitamins and supplements
- If you're aiming to try local cuisine, be sure to check out their menu first. When you want to know about their serving sizes, be sure to ask the waiter or waitress. The reason for this is that most local cuisines tend to go over-board with their servings, where a serving of one can feed two people.
- Try to also include activities when you're on vacation like a brisk walk, water sports, or a visit to the gym. This helps you burn the calories that you gained from the night before.
- Last but not the least, you should never skip meals especially breakfast as this can cause you to indulge yourself in getting more than what you usually get by the next meal time

Figure Thirteen

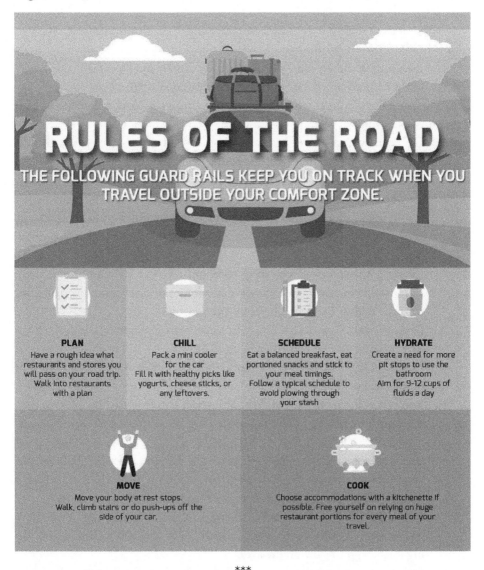

RULES OF THE ROAD

THE FOLLOWING GUARD RAILS KEEP YOU ON TRACK WHEN YOU TRAVEL OUTSIDE YOUR COMFORT ZONE.

PLAN
Have a rough idea what restaurants and stores you will pass on your road trip. Walk into restaurants with a plan

CHILL
Pack a mini cooler for the car Fill it with healthy picks like yogurts, cheese sticks, or any leftovers.

SCHEDULE
Eat a balanced breakfast, eat portioned snacks and stick to your meal timings. Follow a typical schedule to avoid plowing through your stash

HYDRATE
Create a need for more pit stops to use the bathroom Aim for 9-12 cups of fluids a day

MOVE
Move your body at rest stops. Walk, climb stairs or do push-ups off the side of your car.

COOK
Choose accommodations with a kitchenette if possible. Free yourself on relying on huge restaurant portions for every meal of your travel.

***

Slumber for Success

A healthy sleep pattern is one of the keys to successful weight management. Many patients suffer from sleep apnea prior to bariatric surgery. Though sleep apnea improves after bariatric surgery it is still imperative to practice "sleep hygiene "and continue with the treatment for sleep apnea even after surgery.

Chronic lack of sleep is associated with low morning cortisol levels, impaired glucose tolerance and carbohydrate cravings. Increased cortisol increases appetite, leading to night time eating, and signals the body to shift metabolism to store fat.

Work on changing your environment and if you have trouble drifting off try to adopt these healthy sleep habits:

- **Ease into it**: Slowly take your foot off the gas and put it on the brake. Power down an hour before bed. Spend twenty minutes preparing for the next day by prepping your meals and laying out your work clothes. Spend the next twenty minutes getting ready for bed.
- **Get regular**: No matter how tempting it may be to sleep in on weekends, it's better to wake up at the same time every day. Shifting your sleep and wake times pushes your internal clock later.
- **Go to the dark side**: Dim the lights at dinner time to mimic the sunset outside. This promotes melatonin levels. Sleep in total darkness and expose yourself to bright light in the mornings to shut down melatonin production.
- **Create a sanctuary**: Make your bedroom a haven for sleep. Soft sheets, comfortable blankets and pillows, dark shades or heavy curtains make this happen. Banish the television from the bedroom
- **Keep it cool**: Heat delays sleep and leads to sleep fragmentation. Keep the thermostat a few degrees cooler during the day.
- **Impose a kitchen curfew**: Close the kitchen before the lights go out. Eat dinner two to three hours before bed.
- **Ban stress in the bedroom**: Physical reminders of work, like piles of professional journals, and papers to grade need to be eliminated from the bedroom.
- **Ban screens**: Give your electronics a curfew. Devices like smart phones, and computer screens send signals to the brain that it is daytime. Our body's internal clock is highly sensitive to the blue light emitted by screens.
- **Press play**: Tranquilizing tunes like jazz, classical or new age music have been shown to improve the length and depth of your sleep. Choose a soothing music app to slow brainwaves.
- **Sweat sooner**: End exercise sessions three hours before bed to prevent the release of dopamine. If you must work out late, consider low impact exercises like yoga or tai chi.
- **Block out noise**: Night time noise has been shown to increase blood pressure even when you are asleep.
- **Wear socks**: According to the National Sleep foundation heating cold feet causes dilation of the blood vessels, signaling the brain that it is bedtime. The more the dilation, the faster you drift off.

- **Grab a page - turner**: Good old-fashioned reading can help you relax before bed. Unfortunately, the kindle does not count since its light suppresses sleep hormones.
- **Warm bath**: Adjustment of the body temperatures prepares you to sleep. Your core body temperature rises and then falls when you step out of the bath, mimicking what happens when you get drowsy.
- **Practice yoga**: Yoga nidra draws its principles from traditional yoga but does not involve movement. It's a guided meditation to help you sleep, while emphasizing consciousness of your breath. Download an app and sleep yourself to success.
- **Take care of a pet**: Studies have shown that interacting with pets reduces stress and lowers cortisol levels. Pets provide a sense of comfort and security that helps you snooze.
- **Fluid curfew:** According to the Cleveland Clinic skip late night fluid intake that leads to an urge to pee during the night, and wear compression stockings to prevent fluid accumulation in your legs.

Figure Fourteen *(see next page)*

***

Lose-Your-Regain Activity # four: Power Down and Fall Asleep

Sleep experts recommend clearing our heads before we go to sleep. Avoid the blue light from your phone screen, televisions, and computers, an hour before bed for seven nights. Make a to-do list on paper before bed so you don't worry about tasks while staring at the ceiling. This makes it easier to relax and fall asleep.

- Set an alarm an hour before bedtime either to power off devices or turn the screen side down
- Have a pen and note pad beside your bed
- Sit up in bed and list your thoughts for seven days. Divide them into two categories. Things for tomorrow and things for the near future.
- Make another section for thoughts and worries in general. Jot them down in simple words
- Put note pad away, shut off the lights, lie back and take a deep breath. Fall asleep by letting go of your thoughts.

https://go.omadahealth.com

(Health, Omada. "The Omada Program". n.d.)

***

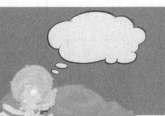

BEST AND WORST SNACKS FOR SLEEP

BEST SNACKS

 - Tart Cherries: Cherries contain melatonin, that control our body's internal clock.

 - Milk: Contains tryptophan a precursor to serotonin, that may make it easier to sleep.

 - Bananas: Filled with muscle relaxants, magnesium and potassium, the carbs contribute to drowsiness.

 - Sweet Potatoes: Promote sleep promoting complex carbohydrates.

WORST SNACKS

 - Dark chocolate: Caffeine and Theobromine are stimulants that increase heart rate and sleeplessness.

 - Alcohol: Although it may help you drift off, it metabolizes quickly, causing you to wake up multiple times.

 - Spicy take-out: In addition to causing heart burn, it can cause trouble falling asleep.

 - Soft drinks: Increased amounts of caffeine serves as a stimulant.

Meet Tammy who is a clinical social worker by profession. She had Lap Band surgery in 2005 and has lost and maintained a 110-pound loss. Here she talks about how she practices mindfulness to keep her on track as she devours her favorite meal of Chickpea Fettucine Alfredo. Practicing portion control and only occasionally allowing yourself to eat a high carbohydrate meal is imperative to maintain weight loss after bariatric surgery.

Figure Fifteen

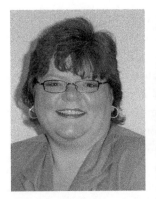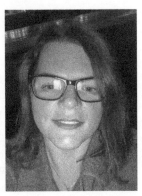

Tammy: I love chickpea-based fettucine alfredo. I do, all that sauce combined with nice thick chickpea pasta – it's the first dish I look for when I sit in front of a menu at an Italian restaurant, or any restaurant for that matter. I guess you could call it my comfort food. Sometimes, I like to add chicken, and sometimes I just like it plain. Ok, before I go too far, yes, I know that Alfredo sauce isn't exactly a low-cal meal, but I don't care, I still love it.

In my weight loss journey, I have learned how to eat my favorite dish, making substitutions and not go overboard. Basically, I live in the moment. I savor and slowly relish every single bite. When the dish arrives and after a good helping of grated parmigiana cheese, I mix it all together. I do that slowly, just mix it around in the bowl. I always take a deep breath and really smell the dish I am about to delight in. That smell of warm cheese mixed together does it for me. Ok, once or twice, I have had my dinner companion say to me, "Are you going to eat that or just smell it all night?" If it's a first date it can be a little embarrassing, but I plow ahead. After it's all mixed together I slowly twirl it around on my fork and spoon – I live in New York where eating pasta correctly is required. Then slowly I take that small amount of pasta and raise it to my mouth and take that first bite. Mmmmmm…sigh.

The first bite is always the best bite. This is the one you will remember, when someone says, "How was dinner last night?" Truly, this is my favorite bite. I take it in my tongue and swirl it around my mouth and slowly savor that bite. I put my spoon and fork down and slowly, very slowly, concentrate on and enjoy that first bite. I chew it until it's digested and on its way down to my tummy. That was a delicious first bite.

Now it's time for some conversation. Then the second bite, again, slowly preparing it on my fork and slowly bringing up to my mouth. This bite is almost as good and I enjoy it again. I make sure to put my fork down between every small bite. Before you know it, almost half the dish is gone. Each bite was enjoyed and almost every time I find that, at this point, I am full. My dinner companion is probably done, having licked their plate clean but I don't care. I've thoroughly enjoyed my dish. And you know what, chances are, at this point, I am done too.

That, in a simple example, is the mindfulness I practice living in the moment, taking in what's in front of you, and paying attention to it, savoring it, making it last. It's about being a thoughtful eater not a mindless eater.

How did I get here, enjoying a bit of chickpea fettucine Alfredo and staying in my size eight jeans from a 26/28?

I grew up as "the fat girl" and I am sure many can identify with that! In 2005, I began my journey to become "the normal girl." April Fool's Day 2005 changed the trajectory of my life, the joke was not on me.

In the days prior to my Lap Band surgery, my highest "known" weight was 287 pounds. I say "known" because that was the last time I would get on the scale. But I have pictures that demonstrate the fact that I was over 300 pounds at one point. The day I had surgery – after my liquid diet – I weighed in at 269. Today, I maintain a weight between 177-185 pounds. I shrank from a size 26/28 and uncomfortably pushing into a 30/32 to a size 8/10 today.

I have maintained a 110-pound weight loss because of a variety of tools in my toolbox. Many of which I will share – however, the main thing that I have learned to use is my own version of mindfulness. And I learned it even before I knew it had a name.

We are hearing "mindfulness" a lot these days about everything from mindful parenting to mindful sex. I am exploring mindful eating from the perspective of an "old" weight loss surgery patient. My greatest fear is that I will fail my surgery and go back to 300-pounds in the blink of an eye. I discovered that mindfulness for a weight loss surgery patient really begins at the "yada, yada, yada…." that my surgical team said, and I thought I would comply with. You know the list – use a small plate, don't drink, and eat at the same time, chew for thirty seconds (put on a timer if you need to), put your fork down between bites, eat small pea size pieces of tough food like meat or fibrous veggies, and the list goes on and on. I'm sure you can add a few more of your own.

Arrogance and ignorance are harsh headmasters I tell you! There were days I thought of my Lap Band in loving terms as my best friend to accompany me on my journey of weight loss toward health. Other days, well – let's just say she put on the black leather and became The Dominatrix – whip in hand to punish careless behavior. Like the day, I went to a friend's Memorial Day bar-b-que and thought I was going to be smart and eat well done London Broil from a paper plate in my lap, with a plastic knife and fork, cutting pieces as large as my thumb. Then trying to wash it all down with a few swallows of iced tea – unsweetened of course! You do see the train wreck heading my way while I so blithely ignored the blaring whistle?

Having weight loss surgery and needing to learn to eat in a whole new way, I had to look at food and the experience of eating – and what it means to eat in a whole new way as well. And let me tell you – I fell on my face many times! When would I learn? How many times was I going to race to the bathroom to throw-up something that got stuck? Stuck because I was rushing. Stuck because I was hiding food that I was eating – and I didn't want someone else to comment on it or take it away from me. Getting something so stuck in my band that I could feel it wriggling around inside me like it was a live fish (see bar-b-que London Broil story above)! Something had to change! What was I missing?

I wish I had known who Jon Kabat-Zinn was and what he was teaching when I started this journey. As with many things along the way, I learned them the hard way, getting my "smart bumps" as my mother always called them. Making me "smart enough" to not do that again.

Chapter Five:

Increase Metabolism and Awaken the Giant Within

"The man who moves a mountain begins by carrying away small stones."
— Confucius

- *Do you have difficulty losing weight? Your body slows your calorie conversion, where you burn less calories on the same amount of portion sizes, and increase your fat storage.*
- *Are you fatigued and tired constantly? Your energy levels may be diminished where iron and B12 deficiencies can cause both fatigue and slowdown of metabolism.*
- *Do you suffer from frequent constipation? It is one of the several factors that contributes to a "slow metabolism". It is estimated that approximately 40% of females and 8% of men suffer from constipation (Nakajima, et al.2018,30123 -7).*
- *Do you suffer from headaches? Tension headaches and migraines associated with an underactive thyroid tend to slow down your metabolism. Fluctuation in levels of cortisol the stress hormone, has also been shown to trigger migraines.*
- *Do you suffer from Cushing's syndrome or Hashimoto's disease? These are underlying causes of an unbalanced metabolism.*

You have finally made it to your goal weight after bariatric surgery. Just because you have dropped all those pounds does not mean that you eat the same amount of food as you did at the beginning of your weight loss journey.

Your metabolism fuels the fire that burns fat in your body. It varies from person to person. It is basically thermodynamics at work.

You might fail to realize that your new body needs less fuel at its new weight. Losing a significant amount of weight causes the body's metabolism to slow down and adapt to the present state. When you try to lose additional weight the metabolism switches to survival mode. This causes a decrease in the daily burn of calories sometimes for as long as up to a year.

What Exactly Is Metabolism?

The word "metabolism "is used to describe the rate at which your body burns calories. Your metabolic rate changes day to day depending on the extent of your activity level. Your basal metabolic rate (BMR) stays steady and is the number of calories your body needs to fuel essential functions like breathing and blood circulation.

The following variables affect your metabolism:

- **Gender**: Males have a higher metabolism than females
- **Age:** Metabolism slows down with age
- **Caffeine**: Stimulants like coffee increase the metabolism
- **Body temperature**: Exposing the body to extreme temperatures increases metabolism
- **Body size**: Bigger the body size, more the calorie burn
- **Hormones**: Thyroid hormones play a crucial role in increasing or decreasing the metabolism
- **Muscle:** The more muscle you have, the more calories you burn, even at rest. It takes more calories for the body to maintain a pound of muscle than it takes for a pound of fat. Inactivity leads to muscle loss and a decline in metabolism
- **Skipping meals**: When you skip meals, your body switches to starvation mode to survive. This results in your metabolism slowing down and making it harder to lose weight. This mechanism will work against you. Your body is hoarding the fat in case it needs the energy later, and starts losing muscle.
- **Hormone:** Leptin, a hormone, helps to normally inhibit hunger. It circulates around and decreases when you starve yourself. Less leptin in the body leads to appetite spikes, which in turn leads to hunger and cravings. Rather than skipping meals or starving, lower your calories just below the maintenance level. You will keep losing the weight and stroking your metabolism (Vetter et al.2017).
- **Timing**: Making changes to the time frame in between meals also circumvents the problem of a sleepy metabolism. A simple action like reducing the bulk of each meal or altering the time schedule of your meals can have an appreciable effect in altering the metabolic rate (Vetter et al,2017).

While some may need a combination of food and exercise regimen modifications, others get by just by shortening the intervals between meals.

In addition to your basal metabolic rate (BMR), two factors affect the calories you burn every day:

1. **Thermogenesis, or processing food:** Your body needs to burn calories for digestion to work.
2. **Exercise:** Any form of activity requires calories to be burned. Any non-exercise activity you perform each day is known as non- exercise activity thermogenesis (NEAT). This burns approximately 100-800 calories per day.

Any additional exercise will burn additional calories which can make a big difference (Levine et al.2006,729-36).

Boosting one's metabolism is the holy grail of every weight loss diet in the market. Eating more often speeds up the metabolism. Three meals a day plus two high protein snacks will suffice. Keep your metabolism humming by adhering to the following time schedule:

- **Breakfast**: Six to eight am
- **Snack**: Ten am
- **Lunch**: Twelve to two pm
- **Snack**: Three to five pm
- **Dinner**: Five to seven pm

Eating every few hours is popular, since eating frequently for some helps them control their hunger and cravings. This also leads to better portion sizes and healthier choices. Skipping meals as part of a controlled eating plan resulting in lower caloric intake may result in health benefits. However, if skipping meals leads to overeating the evening meal, it could result in harmful metabolic changes. Scientific data on both ends of the spectrum have been confusing.

Figure Sixteen

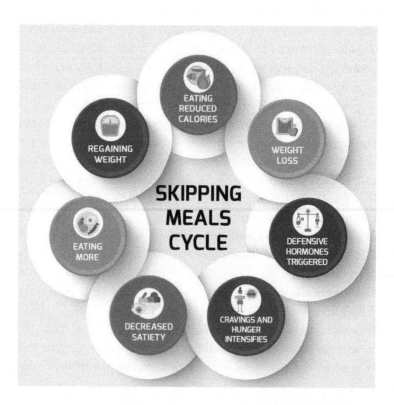

Natural Metabolism Boosters

Certain breakfast foods, in addition to providing energy and satiety, **may** also boost your metabolism. The following foods are loaded with protein, fiber, and good carbohydrates:

Oatmeal is loaded with fiber that keeps you full longer along with lowering your cholesterol. It has a lower glycemic index (GI) and can be paired with yogurt, nuts, and protein powder for an extra boost.

Greek Yogurt may boost your metabolism naturally and contains plenty of protein. Rich in calcium and probiotics, it helps to support a healthy gut, regulate blood sugar levels, and control your appetite.

Coffee is a perfect breakfast option along with vanilla protein shakes in the place of milk added to it. It improves your metabolism, boosts your mood, and helps in burning calories by pumping up the body's metabolic rate.

Eggs are a favorite in breakfast foods that may boost your metabolism. They keep you full longer, maintain blood sugar and insulin levels and are rich in protein, omega-3 fats, and essential amino acids.

Broccoli extracts have been researched, seeming to improve abnormal metabolism and decrease blood sugar levels. Mix it into smoothies, yogurts, or egg omelets.

Cottage Cheese is loaded with protein and keeps you full longer. Pair cottage cheese with fruit or nuts for a healthy breakfast parfait.

Berries like strawberries, raspberries, blackberries, and blueberries may help in boosting your metabolism. They are great breakfast foods which keep your blood sugars stable. Pair them with oatmeal, yogurt, flax seeds or blend them into a smoothie.

Bananas contain a resistant starch that increases satiety. An excellent source of potassium, they help the regulation of nutrient transfer into the cells. This may increase metabolism as well. Watch portion sizes for carb content.

Chia Seeds are loaded with protein, fiber and anti-inflammatory fats. These seeds keep you full longer. They also make a great "breading" for baked fish or chicken.

Cinnamon is a superfood that balances your blood sugar. It lowers appetite, improves satiety, and slows down the gastric emptying.

To keep your metabolism healthy, make sure to fast overnight. (check out more on intermittent fasting in Chapter nine). Throughout the night, the body starts shifting to breaking down primarily fatty acids for energy rather than concentrating on breaking down carbohydrates. This ability of switching from one fuel source to another is called metabolic flexibility and is crucial for regulating healthy blood sugar levels. Confining your eating time to ten to twelve hours during the day helps your body complete a nightly fast of least ten to twelve hours at night. Stay vigilant in eventually cutting yourself off and considering the kitchen closed after dinner (Haluzik & Mraz, 2018,1745 -47).

***

The health of your mitochondria is pivotal when it comes to how robust your metabolism should be, along with your clarity, and focus. Mitochondria produce less energy when they are over worked, when they do not get the nutrients they need, or when they are trying to function in a sedentary body. Mitochondrial deterioration is largely to blame for our fatigue, neurodegenerative diseases, and the length of our lives (Fernsrom et al.2016,1391-97).

Boost your mitochondrial quality and quantity by feeding it and getting it back in the game.

Be nice to your mitochondria, which is the primary power source in your body, since they can either make or break your metabolism. In addition to slowing down the aging process, these tiny factories in our cells enhance your energy, and your body metabolism.

Each one of us has thousands of trillions of these energy factories in our bodies. They are designed to produce adenosine triphosphate (ATP), our bodies' most elemental fuel.

Mitochondria are abundant in areas of the body that demand more energy like the brain, the heart, and the muscles. The health of the mitochondria in your organs is dependent on the current level of your health and fitness. The healthier your mitochondria are, the better you feel, and the more robust your metabolism becomes (Fernsrom et al,2016,1391-97).

As per Bruce. H. Cohen, M.D., a neurologist at Northeast Ohio Medical University, mitochondria produce energy by breaking down the food we eat. Free radicals in moderation can help us fight infection, but when they build up in excess, they damage our bodies, by causing inflammation. (Cohen, Bruce H., 2019)

The main reasons mitochondria deteriorate is due to the excess of poor-quality foods like sugars, flours, and processed foods that we feed our bodies. If you find yourself not eating antioxidants, phytonutrients, healthy fats, protein, and fiber, your body does not have the tools to repair the damage. The pancreas is overworked with over production of insulin, overwhelming the receptors, which ultimately get insulin resistant and are unable to transport it to the cell's mitochondria for energy production (Fernsrom et al.2016,1391-97).

The net result being that unless we take care of our mitochondria, we run a greater risk for several ailments like obesity, type two diabetes and neurodegenerative diseases.

Though a great deal of research still needs to be done, it is guaranteed that eating for your mitochondria will pay off as per Terry Wahls, MD, clinical professor of medicine at University of Iowa. (Wahls, T, Accessed May 3, 2019)

Figure Seventeen

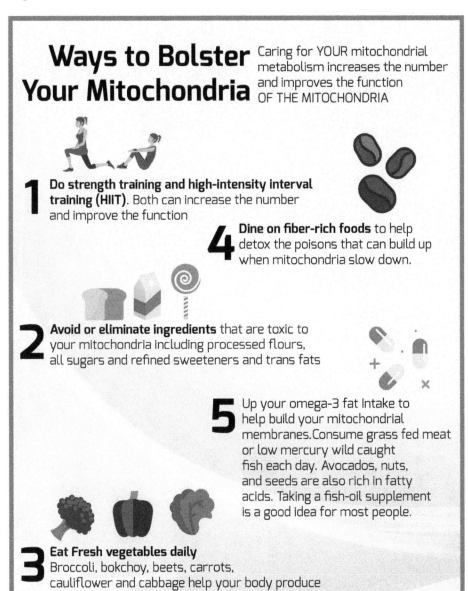

Ways to Bolster Your Mitochondria

Caring for YOUR mitochondrial metabolism increases the number and improves the function OF THE MITOCHONDRIA

1 **Do strength training and high-intensity interval training (HIIT).** Both can increase the number and improve the function

4 **Dine on fiber-rich foods** to help detox the poisons that can build up when mitochondria slow down.

2 **Avoid or eliminate ingredients** that are toxic to your mitochondria including processed flours, all sugars and refined sweeteners and trans fats

5 Up your omega-3 fat Intake to help build your mitochondrial membranes. Consume grass fed meat or low mercury wild caught fish each day. Avocados, nuts, and seeds are also rich in fatty acids. Taking a fish-oil supplement is a good idea for most people.

3 **Eat Fresh vegetables daily** Broccoli, bokchoy, beets, carrots, cauliflower and cabbage help your body produce glutathione, a master oxidant.

***

Certain foods sabotage your body's calorie burning powers. Your endocrine system and your hormone balance predominantly control your metabolism. Any food that disturbs this, throws your metabolism for a loop.

Figure Eighteen

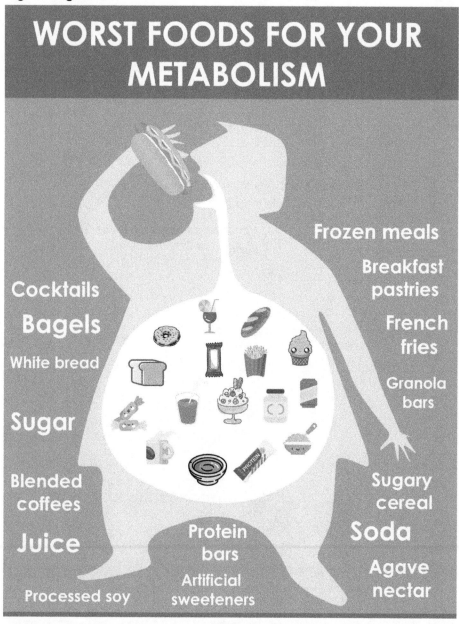

WORST FOODS FOR YOUR METABOLISM

Frozen meals

Breakfast pastries

Cocktails

Bagels

French fries

White bread

Granola bars

Sugar

Blended coffees

Sugary cereal

Juice

Protein bars

Soda

Processed soy

Artificial sweeteners

Agave nectar

***

Constipation is a very common condition after bariatric surgery. When the body has trouble eliminating, it reduces the metabolism and makes it frustrating to lose weight. It is estimated that 40% of females and 8% of males suffer from constipation (Nakajima et al, 2018,30123 -7).

The Unspoken Journey

Constipation after bariatric surgery is "a shift from one's normal routine and frequency." You will most likely have a new normal when it comes to going to the bathroom. If before surgery, you went each morning to the bathroom, after surgery, you may be going only every other day or every two to three days. **Always consult with your doctor before beginning any specific treatment for constipation**. Depending on the severity of constipation, your doctor may have a different recommendation that determines appropriate treatment.

Constipation creates a sluggish digestive system that favors a microbiome better suited for fat gain than fat burning. Along with slow passage of food, the absorption of vitamin B12 is also slowed down (Nakajima et al.2018,30123 -7).

Remember prevention is better than cure. Once you are already constipated, taking Metamucil, flax seeds, or fiber supplements, will be of no help. Adding fiber once you are constipated is like adding sawdust to a sink that is already clogged.

In most cases, constipation after weight loss surgery is caused by the following:
- Reduction in food and drink consumption after surgery
- Taking a prescribed iron supplement
- Taking medications such as chronic pain meds or antidepressants
- Having weak abdominal muscles
- Using narcotic pain medications during the early post-op period. (Discontinue these medications as soon as possible after surgery as to not contribute to constipation.)
- Inadequate fluid intake
- Avoiding diuretics such as coffee that offers caffeine
- Lack of adequate exercise
- Lack of fiber intake
- Eating foods that increase constipation like cheese, peanut butter, and bananas
- Using enemas or taking laxatives frequently
- Ignoring the urge to go

Way to Go

When food enters the body, it goes through a journey that is rarely discussed in company. The last stop is "the urge to go." Here is what happens during the bariatric food "voyage."

Constipation occurs more commonly after lap band, gastric sleeve, and gastric bypass and is less likely with duodenal switch, although it may occur in rare cases with duodenal switch.

Figure Nineteen

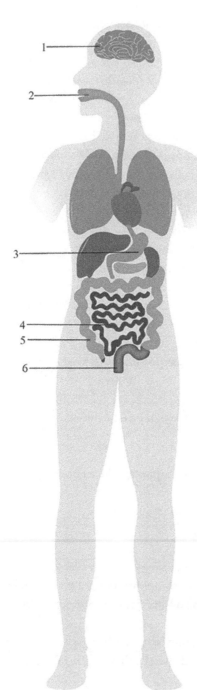

1. Brain
2. Mouth
3. Stomach Pouch
4. Small Intestine
5. Colon or Large Intestine
6. Rectum

1. **The Brain Starts the Digestive Process**

As soon as you start thinking about food, a process called "cephalic digestion" starts. Even before your first bite, digestive enzymes are released. When your mouth starts watering, the stomach pouch readies itself, while your brain stimulates the appetite. Skipping this first stage, where you gobble up your food without chewing it well, or mindlessly eating leads to indigestion of the meal.

2. **The Mouth Follows Next**

Chewing your food well after bariatric surgery helps in assimilating the contents of what you eat. Breaking down the food particles and mixing them with saliva, prompts the digestive enzymes to act on the tiny bites of food. Not chewing enough or eating too fast leads to overeating which in turn impedes the digestive process.

3. **Down the Hatch**

Improperly chewed chunks of food pass through the stomach, irritating the gut as they move along the digestive tract. Any previous weakness or malfunction of the esophageal sphincter, causes stomach acid to be splashed upward causing heart burn. Popping an antacid worsens the constipation situation, since that reduces the available amount of hydrochloric acid that is critical for optimal digestion.

4. **Enter the Small Intestine**

Food leaves the stomach and enters the small intestine where it is broken down into macro and micronutrients. The villi (fingers) of the small intestine are unable to break down and absorb food that has not been chewed well. This food moves through the body undigested and causes large particles of food to seep through fissures in the intestinal lining. Food allergies and intolerances are triggered which further add to the constipation woes.

5. **Into the Colon**

Food has become a bolus (gelatinous glob of bile, digestive food particles and digestive juices) by now. The bolus starts in the ascending colon, moves to the transverse and descending colon. Slowly the bolus shifts from a liquid form to a semisolid form and finally becomes stool. This stool is made up of dead cells, bacteria, undigested fiber, eliminated toxins and water.

6. **Last Stop: Sigmoid Colon and Rectum**

The stool makes its way to the holding pen (sigmoid colon and rectum) till it is ready to leave the body. More water is absorbed as the stool makes its way to the rectum. This is your body's cue that you need to head to the bathroom.

When Things Go Wrong

Not feeling the urge to go, or just ignoring it, leads to constipation. The colon is backed up with stool, which ends up absorbing more water back from the stool.

This leads to stool getting drier, the longer it sits in the colon. The drier it gets, the harder it gets to push out.

A disconnect in any of the above steps throws off your regularity. Start addressing your constipation problem at its root, to get back on track.

If you are experiencing constipation after bariatric surgery, there are simple steps that you can try to alleviate the problem.

1. **Eat a fiber-rich diet**

Fiber is a very important ingredient to ensure that your digestive system works smoothly. There are two types of fiber: soluble and insoluble fiber. Soluble fiber refers to fiber that absorbs water into a gel-like consistency. Soluble fiber slows digestion and is found in oat bran, nuts, seeds, beans, lentils, barley, peas, and some fruits and vegetables. Some types of soluble fiber may help lower risk of heart disease.

Insoluble fiber adds bulk to the stool and appears to help food pass more quickly through the stomach and intestines. It is found in foods such as fresh fruit, vegetables, and complex carbohydrates.

Make sure that you are getting the recommended twenty-five grams of fiber on your bariatric diet. Too much fiber on the other hand may cause more harm than good.

2. **Exercise**

One possible reason for constipation is practicing a sedentary lifestyle. Regular exercise gets your entire body moving, including your internal organs. If you exercise, it can help you stimulate intestinal muscle contractions to improve bowel mobility.

3. **Drink Coffee**

Caffeine has been linked to powering up bowel movements in as little as four minutes. Studies have shown that caffeine in coffee can relax the intestinal tract, which can result to movement in the lower colon. Watch the creamer and sugar intake. Hydrate, hydrate, hydrate while drinking coffee

4. **Load up on healthy fats and probiotics**

Certain foods that are rich in healthy fats and probiotics have been shown to help maintain a healthier digestive system. Including these foods in your diet can help aid digestion.

Healthy fats can be found in nuts, avocadoes, seeds, plant-based oil and fish. Foods rich in probiotics include yogurt, kefir, sauerkraut, buttermilk, miso, and pickles.

5. **Take magnesium supplements**

Magnesium is VERY effective in reducing constipation. Daily use of magnesium will help you regain a regular bowel movement. Unlike laxatives, magnesium is gentle on the body and is non-irritating.

Figure Twenty

HOME REMEDIES THAT HELP WITH CONSTIPATION

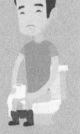

Lemon water acts as a stimulant for the digestive system.

Coffee stimulates your colon. Hydrate alongside your coffee intake.

Prunes and figs

have laxative properties and contain fiber.

Castor oil

stimulates your large intestine. Effective when taken on an empty stomach.

Sesame seeds

consist of an oil composition that helps to lubricate the intestines.

Olive leaves

help relieve discomfort and pain.

Flax seeds

serve as a laxative with high fiber and omega-3 fatty acids.

Aloe Vera

promotes regularity as well as cleanses the colon.

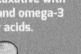

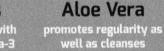

Epsom salt

2 tsp. in a glass of water is all it takes to get the job done.

Baking soda

neutralizes acid within the stomach and causes constipation relief. 1 tsp. added to ¼ cup of warm water.

Psyllium husk

serves as a prebiotic and leads to efficient elimination.

Americans eat approximately five to fourteen grams of fiber a day compared to twenty to twenty-five grams of fiber recommended by most studies to keep the trains running on time (Ma et al,2018).

***

Lose-Your- Regain Activity # five: Celebrate Your Victories by Using Rubber Bands to Count Your Wins

Duration: Five minutes

Completing this skill will remind you that there are many challenges on your path to health but even the biggest obstacles can be overcome by tackling each small victory at a time.

- Buy some colorful rubber bands from the craft store
- Keep these bands either at your desk, or in your pocket book
- Identify an area you need to work on, where either energy, cravings, or emotional triggers have set you off
- Every small effort or challenge you overcome is rewarded by putting a rubber band on your wrist.
- At the end of the day, look at the bands you have on your wrist and reflect upon how you overcame that challenge. This will make you feel empowered.
- Remind yourself to bring them along every morning

https://go.omadahealth.com (Health, Omada."The Omada Program".n.d.)

***

Meet Beth, who feels more confident now to take risks and do things that she would never have done before because of her weight. Her only regret is that she did not do this sooner. Read about how she ultimately learned to love the work required of weight loss surgery patients. Life is work for everyone. You are not exempt, but your attitude is what makes the difference.

Figure Twenty-One

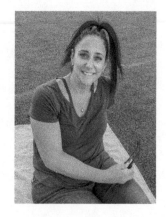

Beth: My weight loss journey began February of 2015 when I had gastric sleeve surgery. I was 306 pounds. As high as that number is for a person's weight, I don't even believe that was my highest. I believe I was hovering around 312-315 pounds. I was so ashamed of myself and just felt like a failure – a monster. I wasn't happy. I wasn't happy with myself, my family, or my job. None of this was my family's fault of course, nor was it my employer's. The problem was me, plain and simple. I used food for everything. Boredom, celebrations, anger (omg, the anger!), anxiety, nervousness and of course, I fit in regular meals. I just couldn't get it together. I was going down the rabbit hole following emotions and food. It needed to end.

My surgeon told me like it was. He was very matter of fact about what was going to happen and that he didn't think I was going to go through with the surgery. I left his office completely beside myself. I cried all the way home and cried for the next week. This man didn't even know me! Who was he to tell me what I would and would not accomplish? Well, after all the tears and avoiding talking about this to anyone, just stewing in my own anger and shame, I read this book about a woman who had gastric sleeve surgery, lost a hundred pounds and was completely happy. I wanted to be her. I wanted my life back. My surgeon was going to be the conduit through which I was going to achieve what I thought was unachievable. I had the surgery and I never looked back. With the help and support of my loving husband, children, friends, co-workers, my nutritionist, and my surgeon I lost 100 pounds. By Christmas of 2015 I had lost fifteen more pounds for a total of 115 pounds. in just over a year. And honestly, as hard as I worked to stay ahead of any weight gain, losing the weight was an easier process than I thought. It was a lot of work, but I was never overwhelmed in the process.

My life is very different now. I plan most of my meals in advance and if I only have time to grab something quickly, I choose a protein drink. I no longer watch morning television – I'm at the gym. I train with a trainer three times a week for thirty minutes. On these days, I tack on thirty minutes of cardio (usually the treadmill or elliptical machine). On the days, I don't workout with my trainer, I do thirty minutes of cardio by myself. I've always gone to the gym but now I work out harder and smarter. My form and endurance are much better. I've seen results from all the hard work. There are some days I ride my bike or walk for two miles. I need to work out. I can't maintain or lose weight just by dieting alone. That's not the way my body works.

During the weight loss process I realized what foods my body can tolerate and what foods I need to avoid. Hamburgers are pretty much intolerable for me. I try to avoid them when I can or I have just a couple of bites. One of my biggest hurdles was lunch of all things. I used to have breakfast, drop my kids off at school, and come back and eat whatever was in the cabinets. I would just graze all morning. By the time lunch came around I didn't want it. I've learned that I must have three meals a day and can't skip any.

I've found new lunch meals that I like and look forward to. I never thought I would say that. I make mini quiches, salads with shaved Brussel sprouts and sunflower seeds, lettuce, and cold cut wraps. I utilize leftover protein from the night before. I would have never done that in the past! For any meal, I make sure that protein is the star of the show. Vegetables are always a part of my meals but not before protein.

Chocolate is a big part of my life. I do crave it. I have found several protein bars that have chocolate that I absolutely love! These bars help me get through the cravings. I look forward to them and think of them as a treat. I'm mindful of portion control because I do experience minor reflux if I eat too much. It's not a feeling I enjoy, so I make sure to look for the signs that I had enough – for example, my nose either runs or gets very stuffy. I sometimes sneeze. I try to take a break from eating at some point and decide if I'm still hungry to continue or if I'm done.

During the summer, that just passed, I had the excess skin removed from my stomach and inner and outer thighs. I was starting to feel down about myself again this past year because of the excess skin. I felt I had worked so hard and yet this skin wasn't going anywhere. I'm ecstatic with the results. I've never looked like this even in my thinnest days. Yes, it was a lot of money. Yes, this was something I would have never considered in the past. But I came to the realization that I'm worth it and I like myself happy. I don't like me anxious and angry. Because of the weight loss accomplishment and the excess skin removal, I won't go back to the person I was five years ago. I don't want to. The very thought of shopping for clothes that really don't look good but function because they happen to fit or being told "the hairstyle is nice but not really for you" or my all-time favorite, "I like the way that looks on you," is not something I want to revisit. I'm proud of the work I put into my overall health and wellbeing.

I'm grateful for this second chance and hope to make the most of it however I can.

Chapter Six:
Grazing, Picking, and Nibbling

"We are all in the gutter. But some of us are looking at the stars."
- Oscar Wilde

Constant grazing boosts your metabolism is a popular weight loss myth. The exact opposite of this is true. Eating constantly throughout the day for no rhyme or reason interferes with burning of your fat stores.

Actually, grazing, picking, or nibbling, prevents your body from burning fat. Constant eating leads to insulin being released consistently in your body putting it in a constant "absorptive phase." This basically means that the insulin in your body starts storing sugar, preventing the other enzymes in your body from moving on from sugar to breaking down fat. The goal of burning fat is to be in a "post absorptive phase" and use your energy sources for sustenance. Grazing does not do that. (Leahey et al,2012,84-91).

In addition, it also makes it tough to keep the necessary track of what you are eating to ensure the right combination of protein, carbohydrates, and fat. Psychologically, the brain is not satisfied with nibbling bites here and there, causing you to overeat later to make up for it. The bottom line is to eat three portion-controlled meals, with the first snack between breakfast and lunch and the second between lunch and dinner. In this manner, your body burns fat and utilizes your energy stores.

New research suggests that grazing especially in the late evening hours could prevent you from losing weight. This could be because the snacks we indulge in at night tend to be less healthy. Ice cream and potato chips munched mindlessly while watching television are metabolically undesirable (Ahmed et al,2018,3321-32).

The more you cut back on meals to make up for snacking, the hungrier you get between meals and the more you snack. Before you know it, grazing becomes a norm in your life. When you see the weight, start coming back, you start wondering, "if you can gain weight just by grazing small amounts all day, how much more weight would you gain if you ate regular meals? This makes you think to just skip meals and continue to snack. You start getting terrified of feeling full.

Grazing makes eating look complicated and sets you up for failure. When you stop grazing, you start meeting your body's needs. Instead of being preoccupied with constant hunger and guilt, you start becoming grateful to be in the present, start concentrating on your surroundings and getting on with your weight loss journey.

To stop grazing, build your meal before it begins

1. This gives you a better picture of what you have on your plate
2. See where you can improve by increasing protein, and fiber
3. Discover the portion sizes you need to sustain yourself till the next meal
4. Brush your teeth after dinner
5. Focus on other interests between meals

Figure Twenty-Two

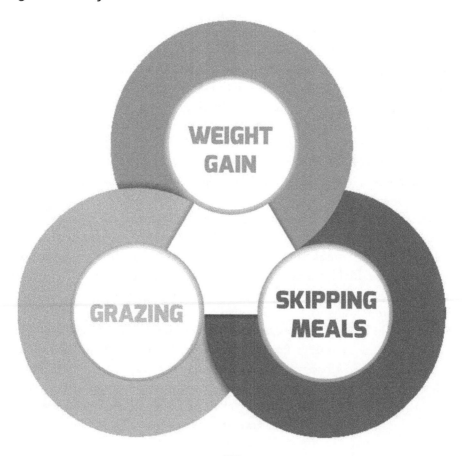

***

Eat O' Clock: Are You Eating the Right Food at the Right Time?

Kathie Swift, MS, RDN, Education Director for the "Food as Medicine" training program at The Center for Mind-Body Medicine, and author of *The Swift Diet*, writes that many stagger through the day time hours, fueling themselves with caffeine and sugar from their favorite coffee shop. This is followed by an evening of overeating and snacking perpetuating this cycle of exhaustion. (Swift, K, et al.2015).

Seven am. scenario: Early Morning Blah

Cortisol levels may be high which trigger cravings for sugar and starch. Avoid breakfast choices that are high in sugar and starch because this will trigger an erratic cycle of energy as your sugar levels spike and fall. Stop this cycle with a breakfast that is built on protein, healthy fat, and fiber. In addition to regulating cortisol levels, it will restore blood sugars to normal levels.

Ten am. scenario: Mid-Morning Roller Coaster

You are absolutely wired after your doughnut and extra-large coffee. Around mid-morning, your energy levels plummet. Insulin has pulled the excess sugar out of your blood stream and you find yourself on an energy rollercoaster.

Rather than giving in to your cravings, reach for snacks like raw veggies, unsalted nuts, or edamame. While the protein will elevate and level off your blood sugar, the fiber will prevent reabsorption in your gut, stabilizing levels.

Two pm. scenario: Post-Lunch Slump

You think you have been good at lunch and had a salad with salad dressing. Or maybe you had pasta. Either way cortisol levels start dropping between two to four pm. Eating a low protein lunch exacerbates the afternoon lethargy. Next day aim for a salad with protein (chicken), fiber, and healthy fats (olives), or a hearty bean soup with veggies and an apple on the side. Both would be better choices.

Six pm. scenario: Not So Happy Hour

You walk into the front door stressed with both cortisol and adrenaline levels well into the final descent of the day. You indulge in alcohol and salty snacks and set yourself into a destructive pattern. If you have not been drinking fluids all day, drink a tall glass of water when you get home. Enjoy a handful of nuts, or half an avocado if you really cannot wait until dinner time.

Ten pm. scenario: Late-Night Noshing

It's almost time for bed, the kitchen is closed but the ice-cream sitting in the freezer keeps calling your name. At this point, as per Swift, your cortisol levels should be in low gear. Any late-night snacking, leads to a spike in insulin levels, interfering with the cortisol dip you need to sleep. According to a study in the journal *Nutrients* a modest 150 calorie protein snack like a couple of raw protein balls or few ounces of cottage cheese consumed around thirty minutes before bed may help protein synthesis and boost metabolism. (Swift, K, et al.2015).

***

High levels of cortisol cause overeating which in turn can become a habit. This raises insulin levels, decreases blood sugar, and causes cravings for sugary, fatty foods. Eating is a source of solace for most people during stressful times.

The bottom line is:

More Stress ⇨ Increased cortisol levels ⇨ Increased appetite ⇨ More fat

The Importance of Cortisol Gone Rogue

Cortisol, also known as the "stress hormone" is produced by the adrenal glands when we are stressed or under pressure. The pituitary gland acts as a gate keeper and decides how much cortisol needs to be released to help you fight stress. It is a beautifully designed alarm system, until it starts to dysfunction.

Being in a constant state of stress triggers the cortisol levels to run amok. This contributes to various problems after bariatric surgery. You sleep less, start craving food, become too fatigued to prep your meals or exercise, and then you experience weight regain. Being in a state of chronic stress puts your cortisol levels in overdrive.

As per Sara Gottfried, MD, author of *The Hormone Reset Diet*, cortisol that is optimally performing follows the "cortisol curve" where it is high in the morning and gradually tapers off during the day, just in time for bed. When your body is chronically stressed, the cortisol curve turns into a rollercoaster. Over time, rogue cortisol wreaks havoc on your body by depleting serotonin levels, causing depression, increasing food addictions and increasing weight around the belly. (Gottfried, S,2017)

Some common malfunctioning patterns that cortisol levels follow are:

Figure Twenty-Three

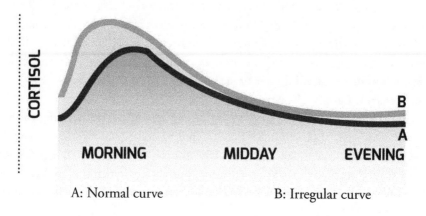

A: Normal curve   B: Irregular curve

A healthy cortisol curve begins with the highest levels highest in the morning before dawn. Normally, cortisol levels are low at three am. and peak around eight am. If you wake up before dawn in a state of anxiety, cortisol levels start spiking much earlier than normal.

1. You are not sleeping throughout the night
2. You are confrontational when you wake up
3. You experience energy crashes and burns around mid-morning (Gottfried, S,2017)

Figure Twenty-Four

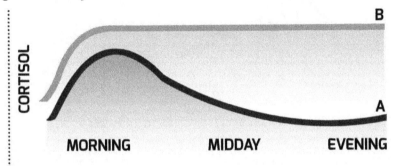

A: Normal curve   B: Irregular curve

Everyday stressors like lack of sleep, work deadlines, and environmental pollution lead to cortisol spikes. A steady elevation in cortisol levels keeps you wired and tires your adrenals.

1. You find yourself always behind at work
2. You are exhausted and riled up at the same time
3. People point out how fast you talk
4. You get irritated very easily (Gottfried, S,2017).

Figure Twenty-Five

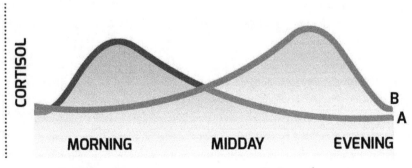

A: Normal curve   B: Irregular curve

If you find yourself arguing at nine pm. or training heavily at the gym in the evening, your cortisol levels are spiking at night. This is the opposite of what you want it to be. This could be due to:

1. You find it impossible to fall asleep
2. You feel argumentative or worried in the evenings (Gottfried, S,2017)

Figure Twenty-Six

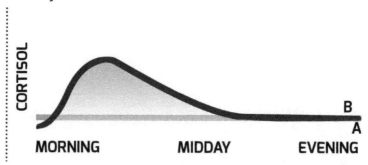

A: Normal curve   B: Irregular curve

After a period of staying elevated, cortisol levels drop off completely. This signals exhaustion of the adrenals. This could be due to prolonged stress, inadequate sleep, and lack of rest. Some common indicators are:

1. You need coffee or intense exercise to wake you up, but it still does not last
2. You tend to fall asleep anywhere
3. You drag through each day, even with plenty of sleep (Gottfried, S,2017)

***

Am I Really Hungry?

Being hungry all the time after bariatric surgery is a death sentence for any weight loss journey.

- *Am I really hungry?*
- *Am I allowed to snack?*
- *Should I chew a piece of gum instead?*
- *What's in a bite?*
- *Should I brush my teeth?*
- *I'm standing and picking, does that count?*
- *What does hunger actually feel like?*
- *Am I procrastinating?*

Do the above questions pass through your mind at some point during the day? The question is what to do about it. For those of you who struggle with the never-ending voices in your head that seems to tell you that you are hungry all the time, running through the flow chart below will clue you into whether the physical evidence for hunger is there.

Figure Twenty-Seven

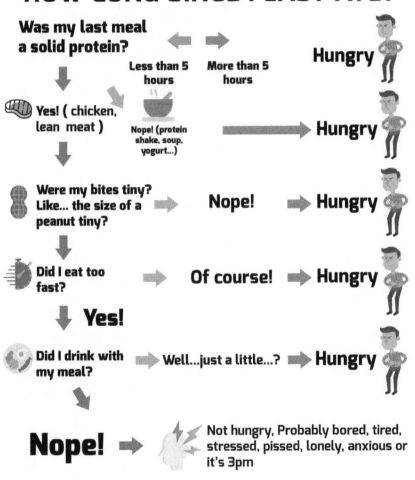

***

Overdoing the GOOD Snacks

"Fruit is a healthy snack"

"Fruit is the perfect mid-morning and after dinner snack"

"Fruit has vitamins and minerals"

"Eating fruit prevents constipation"

Many take the above expressions as an excuse to go overboard on fruit in the name of health.

Are you snacking on too much fruit?

- Your post-operative bariatric habits cause you to follow your new snacking regimen, but replacing it with an overload of fruit is not the answer.
- Fruit might be natural but it still contains fructose and consuming too much of it can create havoc in the insulin department.
- Though fruit is a healthier alternative to sugary desserts, you might be eating too many carbohydrates to allow your body to lose the weight.
- A banana packs almost the same number of carbs as two slices of white bread. A fruit by itself as a snack might keep you satiated for around thirty minutes or so, but adding a protein to it like yogurt or cheese will keep you full longer.
- The fructose from fruit does not trigger the release of leptin (satiety hormone) but instead triggers ghrelin (hunger hormone).
- Eating fruit makes you want to eat more fruit.

Are you snacking on too many nuts?

- Nuts might be low carb, and a healthy source of fat, but that does not mean it is time to overdo it.
- Stick to portion sizes and do not indulge in half the bag.
- Nuts do pile on the pounds if you crunch away mindlessly.
- Many nuts also have an off-balance ratio between omega- 6 and omega- 3, which does not help you either.
- Harvard medical school experts recommend that when you add nuts to your diet, subtract an equivalent number of calories for the rest of the day.

Are you skipping the fat?

- Most bariatric patients believe fat is evil. While some might be, adding healthy fats like avocado, olives, chia seeds and coconut to your diet helps you fight fat.

Are you eating too much healthy fat?

- Quantity is still an issue after bariatric surgery. Being too liberal with your drizzle oil, or eating too many nuts and avocadoes can cause frustration with losing the regained weight.

- Dietary fats have more than twice the calories per gram than protein or carbohydrates do.

It is not the fat by itself but the combination of combining healthy fats with processed carbs and sugars that influences the metabolism and increases inflammation.

***

Lose-Your-Regain Activity # six: Plan and Pack Your Snacks For Seven Days

Duration: Sixty minutes

Prepping ahead is an effective way of reducing or eliminating unhealthy choices. Stash healthy options at your work desk, car, or bag so you can stay clear of the office candy jar, vending machines, and drive-through.

List some healthy high-protein snacks you like or are willing to try. Some power protein options include:

- String cheese and cherry tomatoes.
- Plain Greek yogurt with berries.
- Nuts.
- Hard boiled eggs.
- Edamame.
- Rolled up lettuce, low sodium turkey, and swiss cheese.
- Hummus dip with bell peppers.
- Cucumber slices and tuna salad.
- Kefir pops.
- Lentil patties.

Review and pick your snacks for the next five days. Add the snacks to your shopping list. Prep your snacks ahead of time, by portioning out, washing, and cleaning them.

https://go.omadahealth.com

(Health, Omada. "The Omada Program".n.d.)

***

Meet Tom, who believes that the major step of surgery is a daily reminder of his old habits and the new ones that have formed since his initial consult. He is forever grateful for having the surgery and regaining his life back. Read about how he overcame setbacks during his weight loss journey and stayed motivated. Just like a rollercoaster, challenges make life interesting and exciting. Appreciate the highs for the joy they provide, and the lows for helping you understand what real joy is.

Figure Twenty-Eight

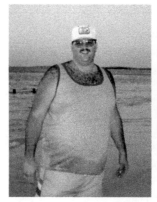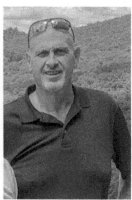

Tom: I was always a big kid! In grammar school I was always in the back of any line. I was 6'3" when I graduated eighth grade, and weighed about 220 pounds. I was very athletic, played baseball and basketball any chance I could.

At twelve years old, I started playing football where my size was a great advantage! But because of my weight, I always had to play with the next age group. At twelve, I was playing with the fourteen-year-old team and at fourteen, with the sixteen-year-old team, etc.

When I was in high school, I was a three-sport athlete, playing football, baseball, track and field. With this level of activity and the workouts, eating was never an issue. As I got older, I got bigger and stronger and my weight increased. However, it was mostly muscle.

Once in college, I played football exclusively since it was a full-time commitment. As a freshman, I weighed 270 pounds. with a chest size of 54 and waist of 40. My coaching staff wanted me to gain some weight, which I did as a sophomore. My playing weight was 295 pounds.

Once my college football career ended, my workout habits changed dramatically, however my eating habits didn't! I ballooned to 330 pounds. I stayed at that weight for a few years, but when I was getting married, I decided I wanted to lose some weight. I went to a doctor who prescribed weight loss medications, and I did lose forty plus pounds. After my wedding, I stopped the pills and started to gain weight again. But I started playing sports again, which helped me lose a few pounds, but mostly maintained my weight.

Fast forward: In my mid-thirties, my job became very stressful, working for a major bank in the IT department, where everything was deadline driven. That, along with working nights, added to the pressure. I found myself stress eating, having two breakfasts – one at work and another when I got home – and two dinners, one at home and again at work! I drank soda incessantly, well into six to seven, two liters bottles a week, not counting for what I drank at home! On the weekends, I liked to have a couple of beers. Back then, light beers were only talked about.

I developed diabetes when I was thirty-five and weighed over 340 pounds. I joined Weight Watchers, lost twenty pounds, and then got frustrated with counting points and gave up. All the weight came back. After another year, my diabetes got more and more out of control, so I tried Weight Watchers again. This time, I lost forty pounds, but again the frustration came back as did the weight. I went through this on and off for six years. I all but gave up! I was taking two blood pressure pills, diabetes pills, and two types of insulin.

Before I met my surgeon and his team, I was up to 370 pounds. and taking eighty units of regular insulin at each meal, and a hundred units of long acting insulin at night! I felt my life was spiraling out of control and I needed to act before the diabetes took my life.

I met with the team at my surgeon's office and they made me feel there was hope for me to turn my life around. We discussed the possibility of two options for weight loss surgery, bypass, or lap band. They told me the pros and cons of each. I didn't really want to go through the invasive operation of bypass, so we decided on the lap band. My surgeon said he thought that was a better option for me, because of my background, and I could always do the bypass later if the lap band failed. So, the process began. I had to lose twenty pounds before the surgery. I also saw the psychologist and nutritionist. The psychologist was very positive and thought because of my athletic history, this was a good option for me.

This gave me the incentive to work out again. With my weight, I had to start out slow, but worked my way up to walking two miles a day before the surgery. I met with the team at the office and then with my surgeon, and we went on to schedule the surgery! I was excited that there might be an answer to my weight situation, yet nervous about having surgery.

On January 26th, 2010, surgery day, my life changed for the better! When I woke up after surgery, I was so ready to start this journey. I followed the doctor's orders and nutritionist's instructions exactly as I was told. I kept those instructions with me always, so I could reference them. The weight started to drop, and as it did, I was able to do more and more. My walking became jogging, and I could do more things with my family, which was seriously lacking before.

Whenever I felt I needed support, whether it be advice or an adjustment, the staff at the office were always there for me. My attitude toward food changed, and as I lost weight my stress level decreased! Since my surgery, I haven't had any carbonated beverages of any kind. In the first three or so years, I didn't eat bread or pasta at all. This was the hardest thing for me to do. I loved those foods, but realized I loved life more, so I didn't eat them. It became easier and easier as the weight came off. Being thinner made me feel much better than eating fatty foods!

I've had some setbacks throughout my journey, including multiple non - bariatric related surgeries and had to have the fluid removed from my band, in case of complications during those surgeries. I did gain weight back, but once I was given the okay, my surgeon and the team replaced the fluid and my weight came off again.

Now eight plus years post-surgery, I work out almost every day and have lost just about 150 pounds. My diabetes medications have almost been eliminated, and I no longer take the 240 units of regular insulin anymore, and take only thirty units of long-acting insulin at night.

I think my desire to be healthy again fueled my motivation and my will power to follow up on all the goals my surgeon and I set for myself. I now have a better understanding of portion control, and do eat some of the foods I missed, (but on rare occasions) and the portions are small, but very satisfying.

In closing, I'd like to say I feel to be a successful lap band patient, you first must have the desire to be healthy; second, motivation and willpower to be healthy; third, follow all the guidelines recommended by the nutritionists and the doctors; fourth, when you do have any questions or doubts, or feel you are starting to gain weight, see the doctor; And fifth, have a strong family support system. I truly believe, although some may think it's excessive, I see the doctor as often as I need to. Therefore, I've been so successful in this journey!

Chapter Seven:

Hydration

"Thousands have lived without love, not one without water."
– W.H. Auden

Incredible as it may seem, good ole water is the single most important catalyst that helps you lose weight and keep it off. Various studies have shown that while increasing your water intake reduces fat deposits, decreasing your water consumption causes more deposition of fat (Thornton, SN,2016).

Have you ever wondered why that happens? Well, when the kidneys are unable to function optimally, due to inadequate hydration, some of their load is dumped on the liver. The primary function of the liver is to metabolize stored fat into energy. It is unable to operate full force if it must do some of the work of the kidneys. Less fat is thereby metabolized and more fat storage happens. This slows down weight loss.

On an average, bariatric protocols point toward sixty-four ounces or more of fluid every day. However, one additional cup of water is needed for every twenty-five pounds of excess weight.

How Do You Know If You're Hydrated?

You've always been told that you need to drink a lot of water. However, many still disregard the importance of this advice. Most people consume far less water than the recommended daily minimum of water of eight cups, regardless of the season. Studies have shown that an optimally hydrated body speeds up its metabolism by 30 % (Thornton, 2016).

How Do You Lose Water?

Water is essential for the human body to maintain its bodily functions. The body uses water to digest, and absorb nutrients and vitamins. Water detoxifies the liver and kidneys, and is critical in the removal of waste.

During these processes the body loses water naturally through sweating, breathing, and digestion. You can also lose water through diet, exercise, stress, environmental temperatures and medication.

As your body uses up its water stores, it becomes important that you replace it by drinking fluids and eating food that contains water.

What Happens When You Don't Have Enough Water?

When you don't replace the water your body is using up, you can experience dehydration. Dehydration can be influenced by different things such as not consuming enough water, exercise intensity, or environmental conditions.

When you are dehydrated, this can contribute to many medical complications including fatigue, joint pain, weight gain, headaches, ulcers, high blood pressure, and kidney disease. Chronic dehydration may even lead to death in severe cases.

Signs of Dehydration

First, check your urine.

One of the most tell-tale signs of dehydration is through the color of your urine. Your urine's color is an indication of how hydrated you are because the body adjusts to varied fluid intakes and adjusts the amount and concentration of fluid that the kidneys release. If your urine's color is a pale yellow or straw color, then you're drinking adequate amounts of fluid. If it's dark colored, like the color of apple juice or you're urinating in smaller volumes, then you are dehydrated.

But even then, these methods are unreliable as you can still produce dark colored urine after drinking lots of water because your body has yet to recover what it lost. Medications and supplements can also cause you to pee in dark colors, even after several hours of taking them.

While severe dehydration can have serious health consequences, mild hydration itself can be damaging. Dehydration can also cause headaches, dry mouth and fatigue (Richardson et al.2009,154-59). You also put yourself at risk for kidney stones when you are dehydrated.

How to Make Hydration a Habit

Make hydration a habit by pausing for a water break. You'll often realize that you can go for hours and hours without drinking a cup of water or even to quench your thirst, but staying hydrated has real advantages. One of which is that it helps you maintain your energy levels and focus so you can work efficiently.

Whether at school or at work, carry a water bottle and make sure it's within arm's reach. It's more likely that you'll grab it to drink water than to go to the nearest vending machine for a can of Coke. When you're frazzled, or stressed out, drink a glass of cold water to help keep your cool and to slow down your heartbeat.

Figure Twenty-Nine

Hate Drinking Plain Water?

 Get creative by adding cut up fruit. Freeze chunks of fruit and use them to ice up your water. Spike it with unusual stuff like basil leaves or tomatoes.

 Count all your water intake including herbal tea and soups.

 Keep your water nearby plus if it helps get an attractive looking water bottle.

 Drink to your favorite temperature. If you like your water warm or cold, go ahead and enjoy it that way.

 Give green tea or ginger-infused tea a try.

 Opt for coconut water.

 Have low sodium broth during meals.

 Try alkaline unflavored water.

 Enjoy sugar free ice pops.

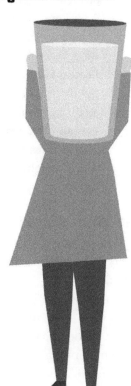

***

Benefits of Lemon Water

Lemons are well known for their healing properties and have tremendous benefits. While in traditional Chinese medicine, lemon water benefits stomach health and digestion, it is thought to be a cleanser and purifier in ayurvedic medicine.

While it is a common belief that lemon water helps, you lose weight, it does not actually have that direct effect. Instead it indirectly helps you replace normal choices of sugary and high calorie drinks with this healthy substitution. Lemon added to water does help make it healthier. In addition to enhancing the flavor of water, it helps you drink more. Pop a few lemon ice cubes from your freezer in a glass of water to maximize the health benefits of lemon water.

- Some people believe that lemon water serves as a daily morning laxative to help prevent constipation. Ayurvedic medicine believes that lemon water jumpstarts the digestive system.
- The citric acid (not ascorbic acid or vitamin C)from lemon water may help prevent the production of calcium oxalate kidney stones. It offers a complementary approach to supporting kidney function.
- Additional flavor can be infused into lemon water by adding mint, ginger or cinnamon.

Healthy ways to add lemon water to your diet

- **Lemon Ginger Drink**: Add one lemon, one inch of fresh ginger and one eighth teaspoon of turmeric to boiling water. Steep for thirty minutes. Strain and drink.
- **Lemon Cucumber Water**: Slice lemon and cucumber into slices. Line your glass with lemon slices and add ice to hold them in place. Next line the glass with cucumber slices and fill with ice. Pour water, let sit to absorb flavors and enjoy.

Eat Your Water

Getting your hydration from foods is a nature -designed smart strategy. Along with deeply hydrating you, it also gives you nutrients and fiber.

Chia seeds

Chia seeds are hydro boosting and encourage satiety. Small black seeds that absorb water more than twelve times its weight, Chia seeds have no flavor and are great in bulking up your snacks and meals. A superfood that displaces calories without compromising on taste, they contain 25% more fiber than flax seeds, and 30% more antioxidants than blueberries. Chia seeds can hold on to water, thereby maintaining your hydration and retaining your electrolytes.

Okra

Okra has a high mucilage content and is an extremely hydrophilic (soluble) fiber food. Adding okra to soups, and stews increases your vitamin A, B6 and C vitamins. It also keeps you full longer.

Oatmeal

Its satiation value makes it the number one choice for breakfast. In addition to providing soluble fiber, oatmeal also contains phosphorus, potassium and selenium. Add chia seeds to oatmeal and start your day off right. There are three types of oats in the market. While steel cut oats take longer to cook, old - fashioned oats have a faster cooking time. Instant oats cook the fastest but digest quicker and do not keep you full longer.

Pears

Just like the apple, a pear is a high hydrophilic fruit. It has more pectin than an apple and helps with regulating the body's absorption of sugar, lowers your cholesterol and aids digestion.

Kidney Beans

Beans can be substituted for protein in a salad and are high –hydrophilic foods. High in antioxidants they can be added to chili-like soups and keeps you full longer.

Oranges

Oranges contain belly-filling pectin and are full of hydrophilic fiber. The thick outer layer is called the pith and contains a lot of pectin in addition to the same amount of vitamin C as the flesh. Oranges are also a great source of Vitamins A, B complex, potassium, and calcium.

Agar

A gelling seaweed widely used in South East Asia, agar is also known as *kanten*. It is 80% hydrophilic fiber with the addition of water. Its hydrophilic properties inhibit the body from storing excess fat.

Figure Thirty *(see next page)*
Infused Water

Create super hydrating sips by muddling one fruit or vegetable from **group A** or **B** in a pitcher. Gently crush one of the flavor boosters from **group C**, add to a cheesecloth or tea infuser and add to the pitcher. Fill a one-quart pitcher with cold water and steep infusion in refrigerator from either fifteen minutes to a maximum of twelve hours.

***

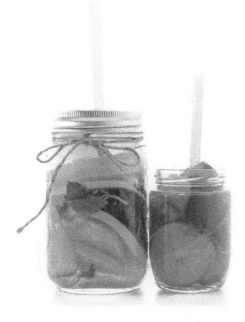

A(FRUIT)
8 watermelon chunks
4 grapefruit or orange sections
3 slices of lemon
½ cup berries
8 pineapple chunks
5 kiwi slices

B (VEGETABLES)
6 zucchini slices
1/2 cup radish
3 stalks celery
3 fennel wedges
½ jalapeno
6 cucumber slices

C(FLAVOR)
1 inch fresh ginger
5 fresh basil leaves
2 sprigs fresh rosemary
2 sprigs of fresh mint
1 inch fresh lemongrass
2 cinnamon sticks

The Sodium-Hydration Link

Sodium does not actually cause weight gain. It causes bloating and water retention which in turn causes the numbers on the scale to rise. When you eat out or binge on a salty snack, you may see a temporary water weight gain of three to five pounds. Exercise helps to flush some of the extra water from your system. While recommendations are one teaspoon of salt =2400 mg of sodium a day, most people consume 3500-4500 mg of sodium a day (Ekmekcioglu et al.2016).

Curtail dietary salt intake by:

- Reading nutrition labels.
- Reducing or eliminating salt from recipes.
- Using herbs and spices to season food.
- Avoid the use of bottled sauces like barbeque, soy, steak, tomato. Use sparingly.
- Avoid canned products.

In our body, salt is considered an important ingredient. This is necessary for regulating blood pressure as well as fluid volumes. It is also a preservative. No wonder salt has been used with other food items to increase shelf life and storage. While salt is important, having too much salt can be dangerous. For instance, you may have been informed not to drink seawater and ocean water because of its high sodium content. Our bodies cannot handle too much salt. This is because the body will swell. This is due to retained water as the body will keep the salt too.

To get rid of this retained water, the solution is just to drink water. It might sound counterproductive but it is true. By drinking water, you will help flush excess salt from your body and hence releasing the retained water. Our body tends to expect a sodium amount and a volume of water. When you tend to drink a lot of water, it somehow learns that you provide more. With the process, it also let's go of the surplus.

Another thing is knowing when your water intake is enough. General guidelines tell us to drink a minimum of eight glasses of water each day even if you are on a diet. When you reach your optimal weight, do so again, so can yield better results such as having more energy and making your skin look better.

Do not forget to listen to your body and always have a glass ready full of water. In this process, you are guaranteed to lose weight, burn fat plus add other great benefits.

***

Carbonating the World

Carbonation causes the sensation of bloating after bariatric surgery. In addition to bloating, patients also report abdominal discomfort due to the smaller stomach size. Soda also has no nutritional value. Though you might have enjoyed the taste in the past, the empty calories contributed by it make it not worth the discomfort. The same goes for seltzer water, beer, champagne, and sparkling wine.

After bariatric surgery, the effects of soda consumption are speedy and dramatic. Assault begins on the bariatric body minutes after the first swig, leading into a sugar induced upward and downward spiral.

Figure Thirty-One

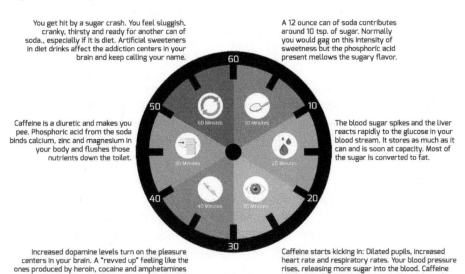

You get hit by a sugar crash. You feel sluggish, cranky, thirsty and ready for another can of soda., especially if it is diet. Artificial sweeteners in diet drinks affect the addiction centers in your brain and keep calling your name.

A 12 ounce can of soda contributes around 10 tsp. of sugar. Normally you would gag on this intensity of sweetness but the phosphoric acid present mellows the sugary flavor.

Caffeine is a diuretic and makes you pee. Phosphoric acid from the soda binds calcium, zinc and magnesium in your body and flushes those nutrients down the toilet.

The blood sugar spikes and the liver reacts rapidly to the glucose in your blood stream. It stores as much as it can and is soon at capacity. Most of the sugar is converted to fat.

Increased dopamine levels turn on the pleasure centers in your brain. A "revved up" feeling like the ones produced by heroin, cocaine and amphetamines is created.

Caffeine starts kicking in: Dilated pupils, increased heart rate and respiratory rates. Your blood pressure rises, releasing more sugar into the blood. Caffeine blocks your brains adenosine receptors and you do not feel tired.

After ten minutes:

A twelve ounce can of soda contributes around ten teaspoons of sugar. Normally you would gag on this intensity of sweetness but the phosphoric acid present mellows the sugary flavor.

After twenty minutes:

The blood sugar spikes and the liver reacts rapidly to the glucose in your blood stream. It stores as much as it can and is soon at capacity. Most of the sugar is converted to fat.

After thirty minutes:

Caffeine starts kicking in: Dilated pupils, increased heart rate and respiratory rates are seen. Your blood pressure rises, releasing more sugar into the blood. Caffeine blocks your brains adenosine receptors and you do not feel tired.

After forty minutes:

Increased dopamine levels turn on the pleasure centers in your brain. A "revved up" feeling like the ones produced by heroin, cocaine and amphetamines is created.

After fifty minutes:

Caffeine is a diuretic and makes you pee. Phosphoric acid from the soda binds calcium, zinc and magnesium in your body and flushes those nutrients down the toilet.

After sixty minutes:

You get hit by a sugar crash. You feel sluggish, cranky, thirsty and ready for another can of soda, especially if it is diet. Artificial sweeteners in diet drinks affect the addiction centers in your brain and keep calling your name.

Plant Waters

Though functional waters like alkaline and plant waters are more in the spotlight, there is not enough evidence to say that they are better than drinking bottled or tap water and more research is needed.

Alkaline Water

While pure water has a pH of seven, alkaline water has a pH higher than seven. The average pH of alkaline waters found in the market are anywhere between eight and nine. While some are naturally alkaline, others undergo processing to become alkaline. Alkaline waters are higher in alkalizing agents like potassium, calcium, silica, and magnesium.

Coconut Water

The trend of functional waters has expanded to include coconut water. The USDA nutrition database points out that an eight-ounce serving of unsweetened ready to drink coconut water offers forty-four calories, eleven grams of carbohydrate, sixty-four milligrams of sodium, nine grams of sugar, and zero grams of protein. Research on coconut water for hydration is mixed and somewhat scarce.

Cactus Water

It is a mixture of prickly pear cactus extract, prickly pear cactus puree, and water. An eight-ounce serving seems to offer twenty-six calories, seven grams of carbohydrate, seven grams of sugar, twelve milligrams of sodium and five milligrams of potassium. Research is still limited on cactus water

Aloe Vera Water

It is often referred to as Aloe Vera juice. An eight-ounce serving offers sixty calories, fifteen grams of carbohydrates, fifteen grams of sugar (including added sugars) and twenty-nine grams of sodium. Studies on ingestion of the above are still scarce.

Lose-Your-Regain Activity # seven: Track Your Fluid Intake

Fluid tracking works like magic to help you with the small changes that will make a real difference with combating the weight regain after bariatric surgery.

Have you been ordering a pumpkin latte four afternoons in a row? Trying to reflect on when and why you continue to make that unhealthy choice could reveal triggers like stress, lack of sleep, low energy levels or a crush on the attractive barista. Tracking your beverage intake will help you take the next step in facing and overcoming it head on.

- Track your calories from fluids seven days a week
- Set specific times of the day to track your fluid intake
- Add one word to describe your state of mind at that time (stressed, tired, bored, cold)
- Review your fluid log after seven days and spot the link between your mind state and the unhealthy choice
- Reflect on what can change for the better and start focusing on a specific realistic goal

https://go.omadahealth.com

(Health, Omada."The Omada Program".n.d.)

***

Meet Vickie, who believes in the mantra that it's not losing the weight, it's maintaining it! Read about how she allows herself to progress, even if it is not perfect. It is better to move forward three steps and back one than to not move forward at all.

Figure Thirty-Two *(see next page)*

Vickie: On March 20, 2014 I had Bariatric surgery, the sleeve. For two weeks prior to surgery, I was on a liquid diet and lost twenty pounds. I had made the decision in November of 2013 to start the process to have the surgery and it was the best decision I have ever made.

Within nine months I lost 135 pounds. I followed the meal plans that were given to me to the letter. From liquids to mushy foods and then finally back to regular food.

It has been an interesting journey. I have learned to cook and think differently about food. My taste buds have changed; foods seem to taste different. Anything too sweet gives me a rush and I get tingly.

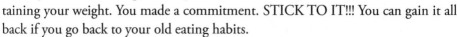
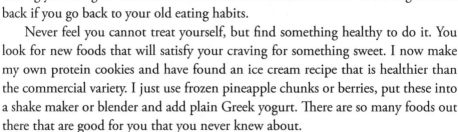

The most important thing I have learned is that you must take responsibility for maintaining your weight. You made a commitment. STICK TO IT!!! You can gain it all back if you go back to your old eating habits.

Never feel you cannot treat yourself, but find something healthy to do it. You look for new foods that will satisfy your craving for something sweet. I now make my own protein cookies and have found an ice cream recipe that is healthier than the commercial variety. I just use frozen pineapple chunks or berries, put these into a shake maker or blender and add plain Greek yogurt. There are so many foods out there that are good for you that you never knew about.

I have maintained my weight for five years by always being conscious of what I am eating. There have been times I have cravings for something I should not have and a few times, I have had real ice cream or a piece of cake or a cookie, but I go right back to my good habits. No one is perfect, but, know your limits. I also have found that keeping myself busy and distracted helps a lot. Most importantly is getting the protein you need because I have found this cuts my hunger and my cravings. I try to eat something every three hours, be it a protein shake, hardboiled egg, yogurt, or a handful of raw almonds. I also always drink water or green tea during the day.

I made a commitment to myself and I recognize that I am the only who can make sure I follow through. I have found distractions to take my mind off eating. I go to the gym at least three days a week and just try to keep myself motivated. The motivation to maintain is easier when I look at my "before" picture and see what I have accomplished. I am proud of myself for achieving my goal and I like what I see and I want to stay there. You must constantly be aware of you. It is not being selfish. You made a commitment…KEEP IT!

Most of all having family and friends that support you is some of the best motivation out there.

Chapter Eight:
Tracking Food Intake

"Change the way you look at things and the things you look at change."
– Wayne W. Dyer

"Food journaling is too much effort and time consuming."
"I cook most of my meals and find it difficult to estimate the amounts of each ingredient."
"I have a hard time figuring out potions."
"I am unable to find certain foods in the food database."
"Meals eaten at a restaurant are hard to log."
"I simply forget to journal."
"I find logging prepackaged foods and fast foods is easier to log, but those are unhealthy."

Have you found yourself in one of the above situations?

Patients who consistently kept a food diary lose almost twice as much weight as those who do not. Weight loss is a numbers game and food tracking helps to keep an account of every calorie.

Food Diary 101

There used to be a British television series called *"Secret Eaters"* which featured overweight individuals who claim that they were not sure why they were gaining weight. To solve the mystery, the television crew employed secret investigators to monitor what exactly were the subjects eating in one week.

After each week, the big reveal showed that almost all of them were eating an alarming amount of food without realizing it. The shock on the faces of the subjects was evidence that they were not aware that throughout the week, they were eating so much junk mindlessly.

A lot of people have this problem. If you are one of those who believe that you're gaining weight even if you only eat a salad at lunch or a small dinner, then maybe it's time for you to start keeping track closely of everything you put in your mouth by keeping a food diary.

What Is a Food Diary?

A lot of people count breakfast lunch and dinner as their main meals. But what is eaten in between is disregarded most of the time. When you start to gain weight even after carefully weighing your portions, why don't you backtrack on your day. Perhaps you forgot to account for that 500-calorie milkshake you had while waiting for your ride home? Or how about that piece of sugar-filled donut your co-worker gave you late afternoon?

Keeping a food diary helps in keeping track of the food you eat in a day. There is no right or wrong way to do this. Some people just write the food to see what they've eaten, some take photos to have a visual reminder instead of writing it, while others use apps that have built in calorie counters (Cordeiro et al.2015).

A food diary also helps you see whether you're putting more healthy food in your body than unhealthy ones. This way, when the scales go up, you don't get surprised.

If you're using a food app with a calorie counter, this can help if you are trying to restrict calorie intake. Although the apps only put a smart estimate, this is still better than just mindlessly putting food in your mouth.

If you have a smartphone, you can download an app in which you can record your food. There are free and paid ones available. You can choose depending on what you feel is most easy to use. Some apps also feature macronutrient count that can also guide you if you need to eat more protein or lessen your carb intake.

For a food diary to be effective, you must religiously record your food honestly and truthfully. If you've eaten two large slices of pizza, don't record "regular-sized pizza." Exactly recording what you ate will help you in the long run to really be mindful of your diet. My advice is also to immediately record the food after you eat so you don't forget and miss out on anything.

What's the Point of Tracking?

Accounting for every food you eat seems like it's only for people who are over-obsessed with their nutrition and their figures. And besides, who even has the time to do that?

But if you are serious about your nutrition and you want to reach your weight loss goals, then knowing what to put in your stomach and how much of it can help you manage the weight helps.

You'll also learn a lot about your eating habits as you track your food.

The *Journal of the American Dietetic Association* published a report that looked at twenty-two research studies on the relationship between weight loss and self-monitored reporting of weight, food eaten, and exercise. Reviewers found a positive association between successful weight loss and diligently tracking food intake where dietary reporting was measured.

While tracking food is no more magical than using a weight loss shake, these studies suggest that the practice simply forces you to reevaluate your eating habits and dietary choices. (Burke et.al. 2011,92-102)

Okay, so if research shows that there's a positive relationship between weight loss and food tracking, how does this help you?

1. It helps with your weight loss goals. For weight loss, food is the bigger factor that contributes to either the success or failure of a program. Most people don't realize how much they're eating, and what they're eating, daily. When you're tracking your food intake, you'll be able to pinpoint where your diet is failing. Are you eating too many pizza slices?

2. You learn what's in your food. Once you've tracked your food intake long enough, you start to better understand the composition of the foods you eat and what you get out of them. For example, you'll realize what's inside that glazed donut that you indulge yourself in for a weekly cheat, or what goes through your body after consuming a six-ounce steak.

Recording incorrect serving sizes leads to inaccuracy of food logs. It is essential to use exact measurements rather than estimating portion sizes. Precision will get you accurate results. Misjudging serving sizes and portion sizes leads to more -than-needed consumption of calories, carbs, and fat.

- While a small sized banana is logged in at ninety-three calories a large sized banana is 185 calories.
- Two to three dates contribute forty-nine calories while a few more dates add up to 163 calories.
- A handful of cashew nuts gives you 179 calories, while a heaped handful contributes almost 600 calories.
- A small teaspoon of peanut butter is forty-three calories, while a tablespoon of peanut butter is 155 calories.

Figure Thirty-Three *(see next page)*

How Do You Know If Tracking Is Right for You?

If you are looking to lose weight, you'll have an easier time meeting this goal when you have more control over your food intake and eating habits. It's as easy as that.

PORTION CONTROL

I ate only 1 banana

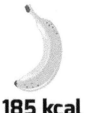

185 kcal   93 kcal

I ate only a few dates

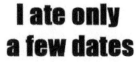

163 kcal   49 kcal

I ate only 1 Tb of peanut butter

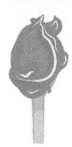 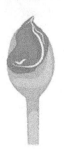

155 kcal   43 kcal

I ate only some cashews

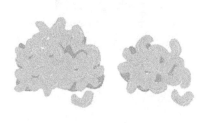

597 kcal   179 kcal

What needs to be tracked?

Once you have a food tracking system or app in place, all you must do is add the food that you eat (both healthy and unhealthy) and the quantity that you've consumed. It doesn't need to be complex either. If you want to be thorough, you can also include side notes like what your mood was when you ate food on this day or what your energy levels were for that day when you ate like this. This helps you generate a paper trail for your eating habits and you find out your true eating habits: do you eat when you're bored or do you eat when you're hungry?

How Do You Start Tracking Your Own Food?

Tracking can be a hassle at first, but remember that it's another skill to learn just like how to follow your exercise regimen at the gym or learning how to cook.

Turn it into a habit and it will be easier for you track down the line. So, here's how you can get started:

1. Choose your tracker: I prefer the pen and paper method, but most people use a mobile app.
2. When you're starting out, ignore the amounts. For the first few weeks of building the habit, write down what you eat without thinking about how much. It's important to build the habit of writing down all the food you eat and then you work your way towards adding in the amount.
3. Log food after you've already eaten. Eventually, you'll want to move towards anticipating what you're going to eat and logging the foods you will be eating, but for now, you'll want to start building up a log after you've eaten. This makes it easy to build up the habit of writing food before working your way towards something as advanced as planning ahead.

A promising opportunity is photo-based journaling, which provides value to the user despite missing entries and is non-judgmental by not emphasizing nutritional details.

Bitesnap is a smart photo food journal app designed around taking photos of food. You log a meal by taking a picture and inputting certain details. It recognizes the food item and calculates the calories and nutrients for you. Though keeping track of what you eat is a simple concept, logging it becomes a chore. Bitesnap is a great tool to identify your eating habits and be mindful of what you are eating. It is available on iPhone and Android in the United States.

***

Tracking Your Probiotic Intake after Bariatric Surgery

Food is much more than its macronutrients (carbs, protein and fat). It also contains micronutrients (vitamins and minerals), phytonutrients (beneficial substances found in plants) and microbes (bacteria and fungi present in our food). Microbiome is the collection of bacteria and other microorganisms residing in your gastrointestinal tract (Guo et al.2018, 43-56). They are responsible for:

*   Food processing.
*   Carbohydrate digestion.
*   Generation of energy.
*   Vitamin synthesis.

- Protecting the body from pathogens.
- Supporting a healthy immune system.

Probiotics: Favorable bacteria that live in your body naturally, and help the intestines in breaking down food and supplementing healthy digestion

Prebiotics: a type of dietary fiber (inulin) used as a food fuel for the gut bacteria to grow.

Foods that contain both prebiotics and probiotics are known as symbiotic foods like cheese, kefir and certain yogurts.

Figure Thirty-Four *(see next page)*

After bariatric surgery, the balance between "good" and "bad" bacteria are altered. This could be due to various reasons like changes in the gastrointestinal tract, usage of antibiotics, changes in gastric acid secretion, and intestinal motility. Any bacterial overgrowth leads to vitamin deficiencies, and malabsorption. Probiotic supplements are not regulated as medications by the food and drug administration (FDA).

The effectiveness of any probiotic depends on the dose and strain of bacteria it contains along with your own unique internal ecosystem. Most studies have centered on two types of bacteria: *Lactobacillus* and *Bifidobacterium,* which are common in digestive health products. In general, you want a supplement to provide at least twenty billion live organisms per dose (Kechagia et al,2013,1-7).

Probiotics are proven to:

- Prevent or treat diarrhea.
- Shorten the length of antibiotic associated diarrhea.
- Treat symptoms of irritable bowel syndrome.
- Relieve symptoms of lactose intolerance.

Four Lifestyle Moves That Can Tip the Scales in Favor of "Good" Bacteria

1. **Play with dirt**: Spending time in the garden, exposes you to microflora in the dirt which helps you grow your own community of helpful bacteria
2. **Consistent exercising** alters the microbiomes in ways that starve off inflammation
3. **Love a dog**: According to research conducted at the University of Colorado, Boulder, dog owners seem to have more diverse microbiomes than their pet- less peers
4. **De-stressors**: Constant stress throws the balance of bacteria out of whack. Practice deep breathing and other self-care activities.

***

WANTED: GOOD GUT BUGS

Start enjoying more foods naturally high in probiotics and in FIBER -RICH PREBIOTICS that help those good bugs thrive.

PROBIOTIC-RICH FOODS

Dairy source
- Yogurt
- Kefir
- Buttermilk
- Lassi - a drink made
  from yogurt and water
- Aged cheeses, such as bleu,
Gouda and cheddar

Fruit & Vegetable sources
- Brined olives
- Tangy chutneys
- Brined olives
- Sauerkraut and its ethnic
  variations-kimchi (korean)
- Sauerruben (fermented sour turnips)
- Pickled beets

Soybean sources
- Miso
- Tempeh
- Soy sauce
- Tamari

Non diary beverages
- kombucha

Other
- Walnuts

PREBIOTIC-RICH FOODS

Veggies
- Tomatoes
- Artichokes
- Onions
- Chicory
- Greens (especially
  dandelion greens)
- Asparagus
- Garlic
- Leeks
- Jerusalem artichokes

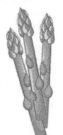

Fruit
- Berries
- Bananas

Whole grains
- Oatmeal
- Flaxseeds
- Freekeh

Legumes
- Lentils
- Kidney beans
- Chickpeas
- Navy beans
- White beans
- Black beans

What is Meal Mapping?

You get into your car, and turn the navigation on to know where you are going, how long it will take you to get there, what the traffic looks like on your route and if you will stop on your way to run an errand or fill gas. This serves as a guide to plan your route for the day. Similarly, you want to plan on nourishing your body with a meal-mapping plan where you design and sketch out your meals and snacks ahead of time.

You must take time to map out what you plan to eat and when you plan to eat it.

Get a new spin on food logging by planning, ahead of time what you plan to eat for the entire day. The **"write before you bite"** ritual might take some effort in the beginning but ends up launching healthier eating after bariatric surgery. The idea is that when it comes time to making meal choices, everything is already planned, and sticking to a script is much easier than relying on will power.

Detail every single bite, down to milk or sugar substitute added to your coffee. This helps you focus on protein and veggies, leaving very little room for treats. When you decide in the morning that you will be cooking fish and vegetables for dinner that day, there is no longer a debate on whether to eat leftovers or pick up pizza after work. It usually turns out that your usual three pm. pastry treat was your lightbulb moment, not out of hunger but out of habit. Do it for a few weeks, to get the preplanning mentality to stick with you long term. Successful meal mapping, leads to a happy, better version of you during your bariatric journey.

- Carve out thirty minutes a day to map out your meals for the week.
- Build your meals and snacks, create grocery lists, and find interesting recipes.
- Use the extra time to channel your stress, practice meditation or some form of physical activity

***

Belly on Fire

Have you indulged in a meal and paid a price for it?

If you suspect that the foods you are eating are triggering or worsening your symptoms of gastroesophageal reflux (GERD), logging your meals and snacks along with the symptoms of heartburn and how often it occurs helps plan a treatment for it. Keep track of symptoms in your food diary like:

- Acid taste in mouth.
- Burning sensation that rises in chest.
- Difficulty or painful swallowing.
- Painful sensation in the stomach, or throat.
- Belching.
- Persistent sore throat.

Heartburn is a familiar foe after bariatric surgery. Chronic heartburn is also known as gastroesophageal reflux disease (GERD) (El-Hadi et al,2014,139-144). While pharmaceutical companies are willing to give a hand, prescription drugs that target heart burn fall under the top ten grossing classes of drugs in the United

States market. While medications do a great job of relieving symptoms temporarily, becoming dependent on them long-term undermines your health over time.

Heartburn is basically faulty plumbing in the esophagus connecting the mouth and stomach. Improper sealing of the lower esophageal sphincter (LES) sloshes up the gastric contents into the esophagus and irritates the lining.

While certain foods after bariatric surgery may contribute to the degree of acid in the stomach, the main problem lies in the functioning capacity of the LES. Hiatal hernia is a common cause of heart burn, when the upper wall of the stomach presses against the diaphragm and adds pressure to the LES.

How can you tell if your heartburn is due to overabundance of acid production or underperformance of the LES?

Elizabeth Lipski, a clinical nutritionist, in her book *Digestive Wellness: Strengthen the immune System and Prevent Disease through Healthy Digestion* suggests an easy home test.

Take a tablespoon of apple cider vinegar and dilute it in a cup of water. Drink the mixture after a meal. If the heart burn symptoms remain, then most likely you have too much acid in your stomach. If on the other hand, your heart burn symptoms improve temporarily, chances are your stomach pouch is not making enough acid (Lipski, 2012).

Lipski offers ways to boost the digestive action:

1. Trigger digestive juices and prepare your digestive system for a meal by engaging your senses. Enjoy the sight and smell of food before you dig into it.
2. Give your digestion a head start by chewing your food thoroughly.
3. Avoid drinking with your meals. It dilutes the available stomach acid and interferes with digestion.
4. Pop digestive enzymes like chewable pepsin (a time released protein digestant available at health food stores) before a meal (Lipski, 2012).

Heartburn Do's and Don'ts

Do's:

- Find out the root cause of your heartburn. It could be stress, food allergies, structural problems, or unhealthy lifestyle habits.
- Raise the head of your bed to keep the contents of the stomach from sliding up against the LES. Either a foam wedge under the mattress or a four by four-inch piece of wood under the top two legs of the bed help.
- Chew your food thoroughly to help digestion, breaking down the food particles, and mixing them with digestive enzymes.

- Even though gum is not encouraged after bariatric surgery, break the rule and consider chewing natural chewing gum after meals. As per recent randomized controlled trials, gum stimulates saliva production, causing a more alkaline environment. (Avoid peppermint flavored gum, which increases acid reflux.)
- Watch portion sizes to lower the odds of increasing the mechanical pressure from the weight of food on the LES.
- Eat fermented foods rich in probiotics like raw cheeses, yogurt, sauerkraut, tempeh, and kombucha
- Indulge in ancient culinary traditions with your meals to stop heartburn before it starts. Nibble on shavings of pickled ginger, or savor an *umeboshi* plum (a pickled fruit found in Asian health food stores).
- Add more vegetables and fruit to keep things moving. Goat's milk dairy products contain less fat than cow's milk and are more digestible.
- Processed foods are filled with hidden ingredients that do not agree with GERD. Eliminate your consumption of them.
- Zap heartburn with fruit: After an attack of acid reflux has begun, research has suggested that having half of a banana acts as a natural antacid. (Lipski, 2012).

Don'ts:
- Stop wearing constrictive clothing that puts pressure on your abdomen
- Don't go to the gym on a full stomach. Vigorous exercises induce acid reflux.
- Don't eat or drink anything that irritates the esophagus like spicy foods, citrus juices, and tomato juice.
- Don't go to bed within two to three hours of eating. Gravity is your friend and you need plenty of time for stomach contents to empty before going horizontal.
- Don't suck on peppermints since they relax the esophageal sphincter, and exacerbate the problem (Lipski, 2012).

***

Lose-Your-Regain Activity # eight: Discover the Positive Effect of Tracking Your Food for Seven Days Straight

Duration: Ten minutes/day

Write down everything you eat or drink from the time you step out of bed in the morning to when you go to sleep at night. Tracking will make you aware of your poor food choices along with the trigger that causes you to make those choices. Once you identify the trigger, you can try to eliminate it by responding in a better way. Removing these impulses will create lasting lifestyle changes.

- Choose your ideal tracking method to enter your meals, snacks, and fluids.
- Select a trigger to remind you to track your meals. The first bite or sip is a great trigger to stop and log your intake.
- Have a backup trigger to remind yourself to track your meals on a consistent basis for seven days. It could be an activity you involve yourself in, a few times a day like heading to the bathroom.
- Start tracking right away and keep up with it.

https://go.omadahealth.com (Health, Omada. "The Omada Program". n.d)

***

Meet Emily who has got her health and self-confidence back after gastric sleeve surgery. She made this lifestyle change not only for herself but for her family. Read about how she went through a successful pregnancy and stays on track as she spends quality time with her baby girl. Every investment in your new lifestyle will help to build your wealth of health in the long run.

Figure Thirty-Five

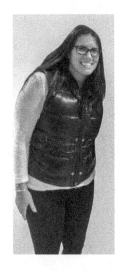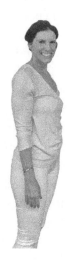

Emily: I've always wondered what it would be like to be thin. I used to dream of the day I could be like "those girls" and prance around in skinny jeans to all the boys' adoration. I never considered losing weight for myself, not considering that my health should come first. It took time for me to realize the extent of the problem. Let me tell you about my experience.

My husband and I had been married for three years and had been talking about starting a family for a while. I couldn't in good conscience get pregnant at my weight. It wouldn't be fair to me or to a child. I went ahead after much deliberation and decided to have the surgery. This decision was not just for me but for my family.

It has been two years and one beautiful, healthy little girl later. Getting to a healthy weight beforehand helped me in maintaining a healthy weight during my pregnancy and ultimately having a smooth delivery, not to mention a daughter with an Apgar score of 9.9! Now that I am the mother of a beautiful newborn, the fear, anxiety, and social judgment I had encountered along the way have vanished. I wouldn't change a thing.

It was very important in my journey, especially during pregnancy to maintain a healthy lifestyle. I made it a point to walk every day. I walked as a way of passing down healthy routines and behaviors to my baby. I didn't have to walk far; the walking alone prompted good thoughts on what to prepare for my next meal. And even though I still indulge myself occasionally, I didn't (and can't stress enough), do not want to ever go back to where I was physically. The amount of energy I have regained and the enhanced mental functioning have been most eye-opening.

I stay on track now with small simple goals every day. I have learned not to beat myself up if I have a bad eating day. The best part and probably the hardest is remembering to snack responsibly. Going too long between meals or when I have a hankering for something to munch on, and then having no healthy options available, I tend to grab whatever is closest and quickest. I still need to remember to keep healthy snacks handy. Also, it helps to keep in mind that there are always recipes to learn and exercises to try to keep up your momentum and motivation.

Lately, my interest has turned to spinning and circuit training classes. I find that I work out best in a group setting. The encouragement of an instructor and the energy in the room pushes me to perform to my best ability. What's more, the people you meet in these classes only inspire and nurture your spirit more. I recently met a woman in class; we count on each other to show up and are determined to keep focused on our goals. Fitness friends at its best! She also has a newborn and is more than ever driven to stay in shape. We lean on each other for accountability and for support.

If I could offer one piece of advice to someone interested in bariatric surgery it is to facilitate and take advantage of the support outlets that surround you, not just in your surgeon's office but out in the real world where there are real deterrents and challenges to face.

Eating is a day- to- day challenge. There are countless blogs and sites dedicated to helping you stay on track; from tricks to tasty breakfast options to easy low carb, high protein dinners. I recommend and rely heavily on frittatas in the morning in muffin- sized portions. I try to stick to a hearty salad for lunch and something reasonable for dinner, fajitas, or a piece of fish. The key is variety. Boredom will only lead to resuming old familiar habits.

I wish for anyone who is considering bariatric surgery to find a team like I had, a team that is supportive not just pre- and post-surgery but one that cares to lend a hand for life. It's important to establish a relationship with yourself too. Ask yourself what your personal objectives are, what do you anticipate changing? There is a great deal to contemplate. This is a life-altering experience, one that I will never regret.

I also wish for anyone considering bariatric surgery the courage to put their life first.

Chapter Nine:

Retraining the Fat Cells. Food, Fat, Freedom Forever

"Formula for success: Rise early, work hard, strike oil."
–Paul Getty

While scientists are hoping to find a magic pill that melts body fat, you can start working on keeping your fat cells trained to protect you from weight regain after bariatric surgery. Dr. Anthony Komaroff, a professor at Harvard Medical school states that brown fat cells do not store fat, they tend to burn it. Increase the number of brown fat cells, while decreasing the white fat cells (Komaroff,2012).

So, what exactly is brown fat versus white fat?

Figure Thirty-Six

BROWN FAT
- Composed of many small lipid droplets and iron containing mitochondria.
- Has higher oxygen consumption.
- Brown fat accumulates around the front neck.
- The purpose is to burn calories to generate heat.
- The quantity of brown fat decreases after life as an infant.

WHITE FAT
- Composed of a single lipid droplet.
- Has low oxygen consumption.
- White fat builds up around the waist and thighs.
- The purpose is it's the largest energy reserve in the body.
- The quantity of white fat increases with age due to consumption of too many calories. and expending too few calories.

Experts are still learning to see how humans can increase their brown fat content. Research is still in the early stages and will be a while before these findings can be used.

Some strategies to generate brown fat as per Dr. Pamela Peeke, a nutrition scholar at the University of Maryland:

- Exercising.
- Getting high quality sleep.
- Exposing yourself to the cold regularly like exercising outdoors.
- Lowering the thermostat in your living and working place (Peeke, https://tipsofthescale.com/51-dr-pamela-peeke/).

David Ludwig, author of *Always Hungry?* refers to insulin as Miracle-Gro™ for fat cells. He points out that eating processed carbohydrates or refined sugar drives fat cells to get hungrier, more motivated to store fat and cause weight regain. Retraining the fat cells by eating healthier "fats" and cutting down on simple carbohydrates, pushes the fat to be released into the bloodstream as energy (Ludwig, D,2018).

Here's How Fat Cells Work and How to Burn Them

The mere mention of the word FAT makes us cringe, but did you know that fats have more purpose in our body than to just make us gain weight?

Let's go back a few years ago. Scientists debunked that a person's BMI or body mass index measures overall health. The authors suggested that having a high BMI doesn't mean that patients face the same health risks that obesity can cause; more importantly, a low BMI doesn't mean that patients were healthier either.

We all need fat, and it's an important part of our cell membranes because this is where energy, vitamins, hormones, and toxins are stored.

Yet higher percentages of body fat (25% and above for men, and 30% and above for women) can be cause for concern (Ho-Pham et al.,2011). This is the case if it's stored in our upper bodies or around our internal organs, which can lead to a lot of problems, ranging from heart diseases to cancer.

But if you want to lose weight, you must understand how fat cells work in our body.

Kirsty Spalding, a molecular biologist who studies fat at the Karolinska Institute in Sweden, discovered that adults keep the same number of fat throughout their lives, regardless if they lose weight or not. Unfortunately, weight loss is basically attributed to shrinkage of fat cells, not making them go away completely (Spalding et al. 2008).

She explained that from infancy to our early twenties, the number of fat cells increase. When we hit our mid-twenties, we maintain the number of fat cells that we have. Some cells may die but our body is quick to replace these cells. "It's as if we're programmed, in a way, to have this number of fat cells," she said. Scientists remain unsure why some people have more fat cells than others.

But these fat cells are not that bad. When fat becomes a part of our body, they become adipose tissue.

Half of our brain is made of fat, and fatty acids contribute to the development of its nerves and its function. We also need fat to develop hormones, which serve as the body's chemical signals between different types of tissues. Fat also provides cushioning for internal organs; think of it like a couch (Spalding et al. 2008)

When we gain weight, we store the extra lipids that we don't use in our fat cells, which then makes them grow. Our weight is related to the number and size of our fat cells. When we lose weight, we shrink these cells but they don't completely disappear. This means that two people with the same body shapes could each have a different number of fat cells, because it depends on how many lipids are stored in these cells (Spalding et al. 2008).

In other words, we lose weight because our fat cells shrink. We don't lose them entirely. When we engage in activities that require energy, our bodies use the chemicals from the food that we eat, and these are often stored in the fat cells. But our body prioritizes the chemicals that weren't yet stored in the fat cells. Once these chemicals are completely burned off, our body moves on to the extra lipids, which is found in our adipose tissue. Burning these lipids is what causes us to lose weight, if we don't replace them (Spalding et al. 2008).

When you start losing fat, your fat cells begin to start filling up with water as a place holder. They wait for the cell to fill up with fat again, when you eat a high calorie, high fat diet. These fat cells are stubborn and hold on for days, hoping to be filled with fat. Once they realize that is not happening, they release themselves and collapse the cell. This leads to a big fat drop on the scale.

When bariatric patients lose a tremendous amount of weight, although the size of the cells shrink in size they do not change in number. Studies have shown that obese persons tend to have more fat cells than the non-obese persons with the number of fat cells increasing with weight regain following weight loss after bariatric surgery. This makes it harder to maintain weight loss due to fat cells sending signals to increase the appetite and store fat.

Here are Strategies for Fat Loss Success

To achieve your fat loss goals, you do not always need to adopt drastic changes to get dramatic results. These fat burners are better than any commercially produced burners because they don't have any side effects.

- **Don't skip meals**. Eat to lose weight because skipping meals can be a factor for you to gain weight instead.

- **Sugar is your enemy, avoid it**. When you eat sugar, this causes the release of the hormone insulin, which is the fat storage hormone. Sugar causes inflammation, which leads to weight gain.
- **Scrap refined carbohydrates** like white flour, white rice, and bread. These can trigger the release of insulin.
- **Visualize your motivation** so you can stick to your goal. You can use a photo of a role model, an old picture of a healthier you, a stunning dress, or maybe of an upcoming event.
- **Sleep for a minimum of seven to eight hours a night**. You need adequate sleep so you will not gain weight.
- **Focus on lost inches** instead of focusing on the numbers on the scale.
- **Make it a habit to read labels** to learn about what's in your food.
- **Make sure you move your body every day**! Time is not an excuse because you can do High Intensity Interval Training (HIIT) for just a few minutes a day.
- **Practice strength training to build muscles**. You burn more calories at rest with more muscle and this is effective for weight loss.
- **Fill your plate** where more than half of your plate is comprised of lean proteins, quarter will be vegetables, and the remaining quarter is complex carbohydrates.
- **When you get unmotivated**, remember why you started, to psyche yourself to move forward.
- **Stop making excuses**. When you feel, yourself trying to make excuses, kick them out!

Fat Burners from the Kitchen

- **Add Turmeric:** The use of curcumin which gives curry its yellow color is a powerful polyphenol. This is a fat blocking nutrient.
- **Add Garlic.** Garlic has a gene which is a sulfur-containing compound that is known to induce cell death in fat cells.
- **Drink Green tea.** Loaded with antioxidants, a cup of tea can be more beneficial to your health in more ways than one.
- **Eat Pears.** A single serving of this underrated fruit is packed with 15% of your daily requirement for fiber, helping you feel full longer.
- **Snack on Almonds.** This might be a surprise for some, but a handful of almonds as part of your daily food intake can help you burn fat quickly, according to a research study published in the *US International Journal of Obesity* (Jackson & Hu, 2014).

- **Add Navy Beans**. Navy beans are powerful fat burners because they are packed with resistant starch. Research shows that eating foods rich in resistant starch, like navy beans, can cause you to burn more fat every day.
- **Dark Chocolate.** Dark chocolate in small amounts is high in antioxidants, and can prevent the buildup of the fat cells in the body that are responsible for obesity and heart disease.

Powerhouse Seeds

Just like nuts, seeds can be a vital part of the bariatric diet. They are high in monounsaturated fat that keep us heart healthy. These tiny guys also contain potent amounts of protein, fiber, vitamins, and minerals. Try to stick to raw seeds and avoid roasted seeds to get the most from them.

Pumpkin seeds are high in omega 3 fatty acids and zinc. They are also high in *phytosterols* which are plant components that keep cholesterol levels stable and enhance the immune system.

Chia seeds are from the mint family. They are packed with protein, fiber and various antioxidants. Studies show that chia seeds promote heart health, increase weight loss by increasing satiety, and stabilize blood sugar levels.

Sunflower seeds promote digestion and increase fiber intake. They are the perfect snack to help you stay full. Packed with good fats, selenium, and copper, they support heart health and balance cellular damage.

Hemp seeds are a super food packed with three-to-one ratio of omega - 6 to omega -3 fatty acids and make an excellent protein snack. In addition to containing ten essential amino acids, hemp seeds contain fiber.

Flax seeds are more beneficial when sprouted and ground into flaxseed meal. This helps you absorb the fiber better and benefit from this rich source of omega- 3 fatty acids. A plant-based protein, flaxseed also contains manganese, thiamine, and magnesium. Check out their nutrients in the following:

Figure Thirty-Seven *(see next page)*

Increasing the Burn:

Why Is Intermittent Fasting Said to Be Effective?

Intermittent fasting is an awesome fat loss tool, nothing else. It is basically how frequently you choose to eat and when.

Intermittent fasting can aid in detoxification, encourage fat burning and improve your immune system.

	Calories	Fat	Protein	Carbs	Fiber
1 Tbsp. Pumpkin seeds	45 calories	4g	2.5g	1g	0.5g
1 Tbsp. Chia seeds	60 calories	4.5 g	3 g	5 g	5 g
1 Tbsp. Sunflower seeds	51 calories	4.5 g	2 g	2 g	1 g
1 Tbsp. Hemp seeds	57 calories	4 g	3 g	1 g	1 g
1 Tbsp. Flax seeds	37 calories	3 g	1 g	2 g	2 g

Credit: (Phillips et al. 2005,9436-45)

Intermittent fasting or time-restricted eating tends to be effective for a lot of people because it is a passive way to lessen calorie intake. And to lose body fat, you need to have a calorie deficit or use up more calories than you consume.

When you only shorten the window of your eating time, there is less chance to eat mindlessly all throughout the day. The shortened time encourages you focus on only the food that you must eat rather than on impulse (Harris et al.2018,507-47). Just doing intermittent fasting can yield results for some people if you're eating normally and not consuming massive amounts of high calorie foods during your non-fasting window. This is common-sense.

But in saying that, you can still combine intermittent fasting with other strategies that can quicken up your fat loss journey.

What Is Intermittent Fasting in the Bariatric World?

Intermittent fasting or "IF" is a way of eating wherein you only consume calories in a shortened period of your day. This means you only start eating during your eating window. The simplest versions usually followed are the 12:12 and 16:8 strategies. This would mean that you only eat during the twelve -hour and eight-hour window. The longer fasting period includes sleeping time, obviously, but you can still drink zero calorie beverages like water, coffee, and tea, as long as you don't add sugar.

For example, if you choose 12:12, you can choose your eating window to start at eight am. and end at eight pm. After breakfast, you can then have your lunch, an afternoon snack, and dinner before eight pm, which is close to your sleeping time anyway.

This schedule may not be suitable for all bariatric patients so the key is to select an eating window that is closer to your natural hunger period. If you typically eat early in the day rather than late, move your eating window earlier. Also consider your training or exercise schedule. We tend to be hungry right after training so what you can do is eat a light, small meal before and after workout so you stay in a neutral, not hungry state.

In the "fed state" your insulin is elevated, signaling the body to store excess calories in your fat cells, while in the "fasted state" your insulin is low and the body starts mobilizing body fat that is stored in your fat cells, burning it for energy. Stored fat is only burned during the fasted state, while you can store more body fat only during the fed state (Harris et al,2018,507-47).

Figure Thirty-Eight

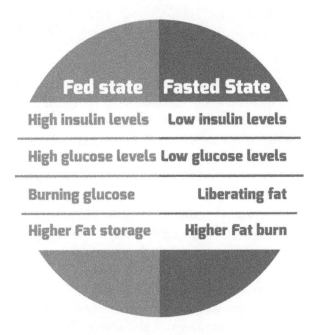

High levels of insulin, also known as hyperinsulinemia have been linked to obesity and heart disease. This also causes your cells to become resistant to the effects of the hormone. When you become resistant to insulin, your pancreas keeps producing even more insulin, causing a vicious cycle.

Figure Thirty-Nine

What raises your insulin?		What lowers your insulin?
High carbohydrate diet.		Low carbohydrate diet.
Frequent eating.		Intermittent fasting/ Consolidated meals.
High caloric intake.	kcal	Low caloric intake.
Sedentary lifestyle.		Active lifestyle.
Empty calories (alcohol).		Increased nutrient density foods.

Combining Intermittent Fasting with Portion Control

If you're already tightening your eating period in a day, why do you still need to control your portions? As I've mentioned, the way to lose body fat is through calorie deficit. This calorie deficit will not happen if you are overloading yourself with calories. Even if you only eat for two hours in a day but ate 7,000 calories in that period, and burned just 2,000 calories – then you'll still experience weight gain.

You must lessen what you eat if you want to lose body fat fast. The good news is, you don't have to manually calculate each calorie of every food item you eat. If you control your portions and only eat nutrient dense food in your diet, then you can gradually see progress.

Figure Forty *(see next page)*

*Caution: **"IF" is not recommended if you are diabetic, have eating disorders, struggle with mental illness, are pregnant or nursing. Please consult your doctor before starting any kind of fast. "IF" is not meant to be practiced long term.**

***

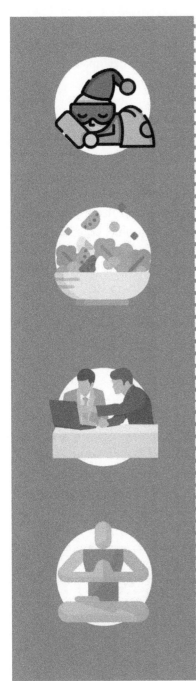

Start by eating an early dinner and avoiding snacks for a few hours before going to bed. Push the first meal of the day back by an hour or so.

Plan your post-fast meal to contain high protein, a vegetable and a fruit. Avoid overeating and eat as if you never fasted.

Try scheduling your fast on a busy day so you benefit from not having to look for food. You will be distracted and less likely to have the urge to eat.

Enjoy your break from food and indulge in low key activities that make you happy. Settle the mind and body.

Lose-Your-Regain Activity # nine: Build a Habit Jar Skill

Are you having a tough time swapping unhealthy habits for healthier ones? This skill will keep you visually motivated by your progress.

How to complete the habit jar skill?

You'll need one clear mason jar and marbles, beads or buttons in two different colors.

- Pick an unhealthy habit you would like to get rid of. Examples are:
- If you would like to eat less carbohydrates and more protein.
- If you would like to spend less time sitting and more time standing at work.
- If you would like to drink less coffee and more water.
- Assign each habit to a color. Keep the jar visible to and let family and friends be aware, so they can cheer you on.
- If you are using beans, every time you perform a healthy habit (eating protein first, not drinking with meals, exercising), drop a red bean into the jar. Every time you perform an unhealthy habit (sitting for longer than thirty minutes at a time, drinking soda or snacking at night) drop a white bean into the jar.

At the end of the week you will be able to see if the white beans outnumber the red ones. This is also a great visual which makes you aware of what habits you need to work on.

Even though the skill-training lasts only a week, you can keep the game going. Motivate yourself by picking a nonfood reward if the red beans outnumber the white beans when the jar gets full.

https://go.omadahealth.com

(Health, Omada. "The Omada Program". n.d.)

***

Meet Elizabeth who believes that her new tool has helped her think about what she is putting in her body nutritionally, helping her achieve weight loss that she could have never imagined. She also believes that if she had to do it again, she would do it in a heartbeat. Read about how she stepped out of her comfort zone, took risks and developed a tolerance. This led to bold actions to create a more satisfying life for herself. Take a risk today, however small it might be.

Figure Forty-One

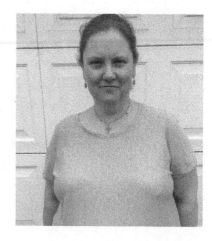

Elizabeth: I don't remember a time when I didn't struggle with trying to lose weight. I was a caregiver for my seriously ill parents from a young age and used to find some comfort in food for a very long time. In November of 2015, I was diagnosed with endometrial cancer. I was in shock and disbelief.

I had been planning to have the gastric sleeve surgery in 2016 but plans quickly changed. I weighed more than 350 pounds, the heaviest in my entire life. I was a size 28/30 and fearful of gaining even more weight. I had been diagnosed not only with cancer but asthma, sleep apnea, high cholesterol, irritable bowel syndrome (IBS) and Type II diabetes. My doctor wanted me to begin taking insulin.

It was during a visit to the oncologist after surgery when I casually remarked, "Don't worry about the scars, I won't be wearing a bathing suit anytime soon let alone a bikini," that one of the medical assistants mentioned the idea of weight loss surgery to me. I had wanted to have the surgery before I was diagnosed with cancer and decided this was the best time to work towards getting it.

I had been so upset after the cancer surgery that I planned my fortieth birthday party right after it for August 2016 thinking that if I succumbed to cancer I would at least have great memories of a big birthday party in my yard with my friends and family laughing and having fun. Soon after that oncology appointment I joined a gym and began working out with a trainer to make positive and lasting changes for my health and overall wellbeing. After taking the necessary steps in 2016 towards weight loss surgery, I had the gastric sleeve done on December 5, 2017. To keep myself motivated over time, I have focused on creating positive habits that are now second nature to me or hard wired into my brain.

Below are a few habits I have created for myself to ensure long-term success. Failure to me is not an option and I have realized while every day may not necessarily be perfect, if I make a great attempt I'm okay with that even if it means that day is imperfectly perfect.

- Control what I can control: I pack my workout clothes in my backpack that I bring to work so I can go to the gym immediately afterwards. Going home and getting caught up in anything else creates an excuse not to workout, which is very easy to do.
- Accountability: I make my appointments a week in advance with my trainer so I am held accountable. This shows a commitment has been made and there is an expectation that exists.
- Celebrate achievements: I was recently able to deadlift 150 pounds. during one of my workouts. This was an amazing accomplishment. When I began working out more than a year and a half ago it would take me four minutes to row 300m on the rowing machine. Now I can do 500m consistently in 2:30 or less.
- Variety: I try a new recipe every week that's focused on my bariatric needs. As the journey continues, I do not want to get bored by eating the same foods all the time and potentially go off track.
- Documentation: I created a rewards journal where I list things I want to do that are not food related. One example is travel to Ireland. Another is to run

a 5K or 10K race. I also started using non-food rewards like acupuncture, Reiki, kickboxing, and the gym for stress management.

- Make it a team effort: I was selective with who I told about my decision about getting surgery. Close friends and family that know, have been wonderfully supportive. Those that are into cooking have shown me how I can modify recipes to make them for my bariatric needs. Some have gone shopping with me and I have been able to celebrate getting out of the plus size clothing section.

As I reflect on where I was in 2015 and today, I'm thankful for the support and guidance from the medical professionals who have helped me, the friends and family who have taken it upon themselves to learn about my bariatric needs, and my trainer, who has kept me motivated during many workouts and who pushes me to become stronger.

Chapter Ten:

Exercising

*"Those who think they have no time for exercise
will sooner or later have to find time for illness."*
–Edward Stanley

It's Your Move: No More Excuses

*H*ave you ever signed up for a gym membership only to realize that the number of times you've gone does not justify the exorbitant fee?

Are your exercise clothes building cobwebs at the corner of your closet due to months of being unused?

And how many times have you pushed that snooze button the morning you promised yourself that you're going to start running again?

You are not alone. A lot of people find different excuses to get out of exercise. Sometimes it's staying late at work that prevents them from going to the gym. For some, it's personal issues, while for most people, it's a bout of laziness or disinterest.

After bariatric surgery, patients establish an exercise routine that works for them. This could either involve walking, light cardio, or strength training. To get more from their workout, it is important to switch things up a bit to maintain the metabolism.

After six to eight weeks, the body adapts to the type, amount, and intensity of exercise that is being done. Patients hit a fitness plateau repeating the same exercise regime, and they stop getting stronger and fitter. Fitness plateaus happen when you overload your body with varied exercises. In turn, your muscles and your system will adapt to these movements. This is the body's physiological outcome. When this happens, you need to create a progression in the kind of load and intensity of the workouts. If you are not able to do it, chances are your improvement will stall.

Jumpstart progress either by increasing the resistance, moving faster or moving in different ways. This usually does the trick.

Turn Your No Time into Yes Time for Exercise

Here are suggested activities that you can do in favor of having that much-needed workout.

Working Out While Working

They say work takes a lot of our time in a day. How about we incorporate a workout while we work? There are many things you can do to make this happen.
Some Examples:

- Walk to get your lunch rather than taking a cab.
- You can even walk the stairs rather than taking the elevator.
- Move around during breaks in your office rather than staying in your cubicle for the entire eight hours.
- Turn phone time into active time. Hit the treadmill or the stationary bike while doing your daily family or friends phone catchup from home.

How to Upgrade Your Workouts

Upgrade one: Alter Your Sequencing

An effective way to push yourself is to change the order you exercise. For instance, if you start your workout by going on the treadmill first, try the rower instead. Rather than beginning your yoga practice with sun salutations, try starting with the "downward dog" pose. This new sequence forces the muscles to get stronger through fatigue.

Upgrade two: Walk with Nature

Most bariatric patients are avid walkers. Rather than walk on the treadmill, to burn more calories seek outdoor routes that force you to walk navigate obstacles like curbs, slopes, and rocks.

Upgrade three: Adapt Different Angles

Experiment with your strength training circuit by doing more reps or adding more weight. Over time bicep curls and squats overuse and tighten some muscles and weaken others. Changing the angle of the body by adapting variations of these exercises helps in building strength.

If you are still not seeing results, consider other factors. When you are slowly seeing signs of a fitness plateau, you tend to become stressed and feel inferior. It is important to stick to the goal and remember why you are doing the workout and the hard work. Sometimes, it is not about the workout but rather life's other triggers, like stress, lack of sleep, and poor nutrition. You will need sufficient sleep to support your routine.

Lacking in this aspect means an increase of the stress hormones that in turn can compromise workout results.

Replace Activities to Make Time for Exercise

We have a lot of activities in one day that are considered unnecessary, such as watching bad television shows or browsing through social media accounts excessively. If you have the time to do this, then you have the time to exercise. Better put down the phone or turn off your computer and hit the gym. Skip this unnecessary activity in favor of a short workout.

- Mark your calendar and commit to planned exercise. Stop skipping appointments with yourself.
- No matter what the day looks like, exercise first thing in the morning and have back up plans for days you are unable to start early.
- Always exercise on Mondays. This sets the tone for the rest of the week.
- Never skip exercising for two days in a row.
- Even if you are tired, go through the motions. After the first ten minutes, you will be glad you started.

Remember exercise is not a luxury, it is a necessity. So always have the "yes time" mentality rather than the "no time."

The Hidden Benefits of Exercise

The benefits of exercise are almost instantaneous. The moment you head into your spin class or to your Pilates session, the benefits of exercise start to kick in. Your heart rate goes up, and blood is delivered to the muscles. You burn calories for fuel and immediately get a mood boost. You could add years to your life just by doing thirty minutes of cardio three to five days a week.

On top of that, exercise will not only help you live longer but also help you look younger and feel happier. Your body also has more energy and you're ready to stay healthy.

That's just the beginning. Keep on reading and you'll discover some of the quick and long-lasting benefits of regular exercise.

What happens when you continue to work out?

As you continue to work out, your lungs get stronger. When doing cardio, the brain sends signals to the lungs to help you breathe faster and deeper, delivering extra oxygen to the muscles. Your motivation is at its peak. The endorphins start to flood in, triggering the classic runner's high.

What happens within an hour of exercise?

You start to protect yourself against colds, flu, and other sickness. Exercise elevates levels of immunoglobins – proteins that help boost the immune system and fight infection.

Your mood-enhancing chemicals start to flood your brain for a couple of hours after the exercise, and for a day, your mood and body feel at Zen.

Even when you're resting, you're burning calories.

This means that if you went on a three-mile run, you'd be burning about 300 calories, and still be burning a few more forty-five minutes later.

What happens to your body within a day of exercise?

If your routine involved strength training, you are potentially adding lean muscle after exercising. After one day, your muscles are now rebuilding themselves, repairing the microscopic tears that come with weightlifting.

Your heart is also healthier. A sweat session lowers blood pressure for up to sixteen hours. You're also thinking very quickly. You're more alert and focused after the exercise. This is because a good workout increases flow of blood and oxygen to the brain.

What happens after a week of regular exercise?

Your risk of diabetes starts going down. The more you work out, the greater the sensitivity to insulin. Regular exercise lowers blood sugar levels and reduces the risk of Type two diabetes.

Your maximal oxygen consumption or VO2 max, which is a measure for endurance and aerobic fitness, has already increased by about five percent. The more regularly you exercise, the higher your endurance develops (Lanza, 2015,3656 -58).

At this point, you're now toned. You're cutting about 500 calories a day through exercise alone. Combining this with diet will help you drop up to one pound a week.

The long-term benefits of exercising

You're getting stronger, and those ten-pound weights don't feel quite as heavy as they did before. This is because your modular endurance is starting to increase. Your ten reps are no longer a struggle with the same weight. You can now aim for higher rep count using the weight that you struggled to do ten reps with last week.

After four weeks of regularly working out, you're already burning off belly fat. You're burning off flab and gaining muscle (Lanza, 2015,3656 -58).

What happens after a year?

Your work outs are easier. Your heart rate is also lower thanks to the regular workouts. Your heart is now pumping more efficiently. If your initial heart rate before was eighty beats per minute (BPM), it has now dropped to seventy or lower. The less work your heart does, the healthier your body. You're also adding years to your life.

Pick a Dance, Any Dance

Different dance styles that will fit your bill, no matter which health payoff you seek.

Figure Forty-Two

If you feel like......	Try	Which you love.	Average calorie burn per hour.
Killing calories and upping the excitement.	Hip Hop	The number of calories burned depends on the intensity of the class. A heart pounder.	**540**
Dancing even with bad knees.	Ballroom	A slow waltz is easy on the knees. No rapid turns. Keep your body straight. Grab a friend and click play.	**240**
Sculpting and toning.	Cardio Ballet	Break a sweat by blending light weights and strength boosting exercises with classic moves from the barre.	**480**
Improving balance.	Salsa	Boost coordination and stability with frequent changes in direction.	**540**
Moving but not worrying about coordination.	Zumba	No wrong way to do it.	**540**

Credit: *Calories Burned Dancing Calculator*. Captain Calculator, 2014, captaincalculator.com/health/calorie/calories-burned-dancing-calculator/

Figure Forty-Three

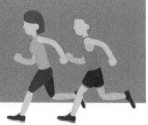

HEART RATE & EXERCISE

Your heart rate is the most accurate indicator of how intensely you're working during exercise.

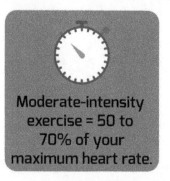

Moderate-intensity exercise = 50 to 70% of your maximum heart rate.

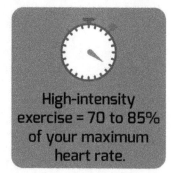

High-intensity exercise = 70 to 85% of your maximum heart rate.

LET'S CALCULATE YOUR MAXIMUM HEART RATE

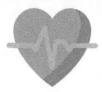

220 - (Your age) = Your maximum heart rate.

If you're 50 years old, your max heart rate would be 220 - 50 = 170.

YOU CAN MEASURE BY TAKING YOUR PULSE...

To measure your heart rate by taking your pulse: Set a timer for 10 seconds, place two fingers on the inside of your wrist and count how many times your heart beats. Multiply that number by 6 to get your current heart rate.

.... or use a fitness tracking device with a built-in heart rate monitor.

No Gym? No Problem

There are many reasons why individuals do not exercise. It could be because the gym is very far from where they are residing and accessibility can be an issue. **Or,** they just don't have the time to exercise because of their work and busy lifestyle. **Or,** the gym membership can be pricey and not everyone can afford to pay it monthly or annually. These are the reasons why others find a more convenient way to exercise. Good thing is there are exercises that you can do even without hitting the gym, and yet reap meaningful benefits.

Figure Forty-Four

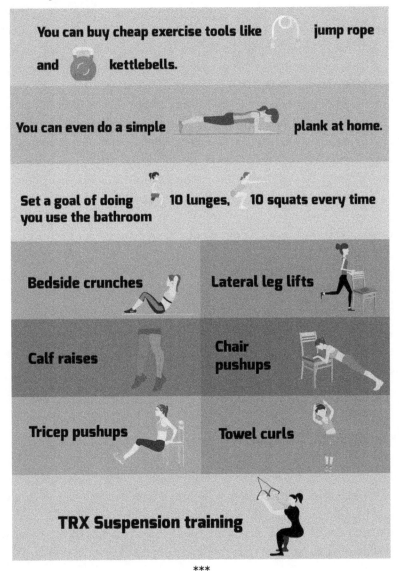

You can buy cheap exercise tools like jump rope and kettlebells.

You can even do a simple plank at home.

Set a goal of doing 10 lunges, 10 squats every time you use the bathroom

Bedside crunches

Lateral leg lifts

Calf raises

Chair pushups

Tricep pushups

Towel curls

TRX Suspension training

***

A Small Snack After Workout Is a Must: Here's Why

You have been working hard at the gym. You have finished a few rounds of routines. You are sweating like crazy. After all your hard work, it is now time to reward yourself. And a common treat after exercise is food. Since your body has lost a lot of fluid and calories, a little reward would go a long way. There also are others who would rather not eat.

When you forego eating a healthy source of protein before or after you have exercised, you defeat the purpose of exercise.

Individuals who eat a lot after a workout simply negate the exercise. They could be adding more calories to their bodies rather than eliminating them. In short, they could be sabotaging their weight loss. If you would rather not eat after a workout because you are serious about your weight loss journey, you could be doing more harm than good to your body.

After a workout, it is normal not to feel hungry at all. After all, an intense round of exercise can lower ghrelin. This is the hormone that stimulates the appetite. It would usually take three to four hours before your hunger returns to normal. Because of that long period of time, dismissing the need to eat after a workout is a big no-no. If you delay eating and just eat when your body finally feels the hunger, you might eat more in the process. As soon as your appetite is back, you might be binging on more calories. Additionally, delaying food can slow your recovery process. It would be harder to hit the gym next because your body hasn't recovered yet.

When experts say, "Eat after a workout," you don't have to overindulge. A small recovery snack is preferred rather than a whole meal. Some examples are

- One small apple with one tablespoon of peanut (or almond) butter.
- Greek yogurt with added fruit.
- Protein shake.
- Two low sodium turkey and cheese roll ups.

Figure Forty-Five *(see next page)*

Walk Away Your Weight

If you want to lose weight quick and efficiently, you could get started on a walking program. It's a low-impact exercise that's so easy to fit into a busy schedule, and can be done by anyone regardless of age or fitness level. Power walking, for instance is a great workout, and even greater when it's done in the morning. Try to do thirty to forty-five minutes of power walks four to five days a week. Then set yourself up to longer durations as you progress.

Shadow Boxing and the Bariatric Body

Throwing a punch is a physically and mentally challenging way to break out into a sweat. Boxing serves as a full body workout for both the upper and lower body. It uses balance and coordination of both sides of the body as well.

There is no need for a partner or any kind of equipment. Master three basic moves of a jab, cross and lead hook for a high intensity workout that can be done in your living room. Focus on form first before you build up speed and power.

Starting Stance

- Stand with feet hip width apart
- Place your dominant leg backward
- Keep both knees soft
- Keep elbows close to body
- Fists a few inches from your face
- Tuck chin in slightly
- Your forward foot is called the "lead"

Jab

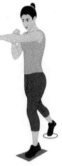

- Exhale as you extend your lead arm
- Turn your fist to angle the knuckles down
- Keep your rear hand by face
- Round your lead shoulder inward to protect your face
- Reverse to return to starting stance

Cross

- Rotate forward on ball of back foot
- Exhale as you rotate your torso
- Extend your rear arm, turning your fist down to keep the wrist straight
- Keep lead hand by your face
- Reverse to return to starting stance

Lead Hook

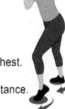

- Plant your rear foot firmly
- Come on to balls of the lead foot.
- Rotate your torso and feet, bringing your lead arm in a semicircular strike
- Your fist ends in front of your chest, with palm facing your chest.
- Keep rear hand by face
- Reverse to return to starting stance.

Combine these boxing moves with jumping rope and pushups for a shadowboxing circuit
- Jab-Cross-Hook combo with dominant leg in lead position for 60 seconds
- Rest 30 seconds
- Jump rope for 60 seconds
- Rest for 30 seconds
- Jab-Cross-Hook combo with dominant leg in rear position for 60 seconds
- Rest 30 seconds
- Pushups for 20 seconds.

Perform a total of three rounds of above 5-minute workout .

To get to your weight loss goals, take short walks for at least twenty minutes following every meal. This helps you control blood sugar and prevent cravings for more food. This also boosts your metabolism. Another way of getting walking into your regimen is to take the stairs instead of the elevator. If you're only going down two floors, take the stairs to and from the destination.

At night, once you are off work, you can walk for another thirty to forty-five minutes. If you're just going down a couple of blocks to buy something from the store, try walking instead of driving. Not only are you burning fat, but you're also saving up on fuel consumption and reducing greenhouse gas emissions.

Figure Forty-Six

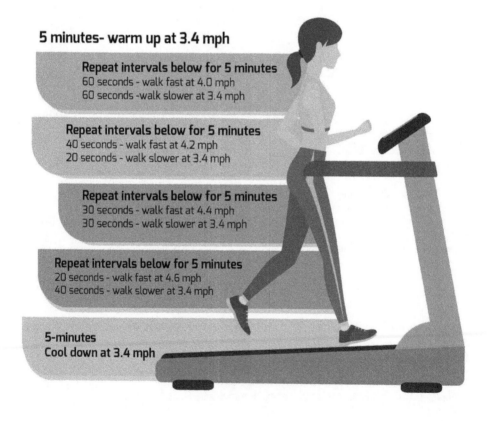

5 minutes- warm up at 3.4 mph

Repeat intervals below for 5 minutes
60 seconds - walk fast at 4.0 mph
60 seconds -walk slower at 3.4 mph

Repeat intervals below for 5 minutes
40 seconds - walk fast at 4.2 mph
20 seconds - walk slower at 3.4 mph

Repeat intervals below for 5 minutes
30 seconds - walk fast at 4.4 mph
30 seconds - walk slower at 3.4 mph

Repeat intervals below for 5 minutes
20 seconds - walk fast at 4.6 mph
40 seconds - walk slower at 3.4 mph

5-minutes
Cool down at 3.4 mph

***

Figure Forty-Seven

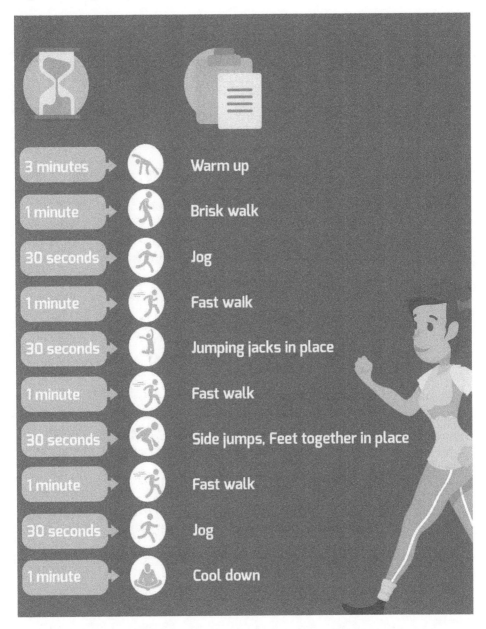

3 minutes		Warm up
1 minute		Brisk walk
30 seconds		Jog
1 minute		Fast walk
30 seconds		Jumping jacks in place
1 minute		Fast walk
30 seconds		Side jumps, Feet together in place
1 minute		Fast walk
30 seconds		Jog
1 minute		Cool down

***

Figure Forty-Eight

	 Warm Up	Activity	 Cool Down	 Total Time
Week 1	Walk slowly 5 minutes	Then walk briskly 5 minutes	Then walk slowly 5 minutes	15 minutes
Week 2	Walk slowly 5 minutes	Then walk briskly 7 minutes	Then walk slowly 5 minutes	17 minutes
Week 3	Walk slowly 5 minutes	Then walk briskly 9 minutes	Then walk slowly 5 minutes	19 minutes
Week 4	Walk slowly 5 minutes	Then walk briskly 11 minutes	Then walk slowly 5 minutes	21 minutes
Week 5	Walk slowly 5 minutes	Then walk briskly 13 minutes	Then walk slowly 5 minutes	23 minutes
Week 6	Walk slowly 5 minutes	Then walk briskly 15 minutes	Then walk slowly 5 minutes	25 minutes
Week 7	Walk slowly 5 minutes	Then walk briskly 18 minutes	Then walk slowly 5 minutes	28 minutes
Week 8	Walk slowly 5 minutes	Then walk briskly 20 minutes	Then walk slowly 5 minutes	30 minutes
Week 9	Walk slowly 5 minutes	Then walk briskly 23 minutes	Then walk slowly 5 minutes	33 minutes
Week 10	Walk slowly 5 minutes	Then walk briskly 26 minutes	Then walk slowly 5 minutes	36 minutes
Week 11	Walk slowly 5 minutes	Then walk briskly 28 minutes	Then walk slowly 5 minutes	38 minutes
Week 12	Walk slowly 5 minutes	Then walk briskly 30 minutes	Then walk slowly 5 minutes	40 minutes

Figure Forty-Nine

WATER WORKOUT

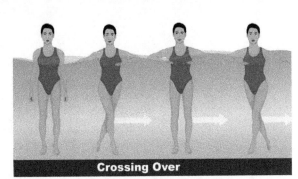

Warm Up

- Warm up by doing a slow march in place
- Swing your arms and bring your knees up
- Keep core muscles engaged
- March for 45 seconds
- Take a 15 second break
- Repeat 3 times

Crossing Over

- Stand sideways in your lane with feet a few inches apart
- Face direction you will be moving in
- Cross your right foot over front of your left foot
- Move your left foot out, returning to your beginning stance.
- Use your outstretched arms for balance
- Next place your right foot behind your left foot. Once again, move your left foot out, and return to your beginning stance.
- Continue this pattern travelling all the way down the lane
- Complete 30 second sets in each direction for a total of four sets.
- Rest for 15 seconds in between sets.

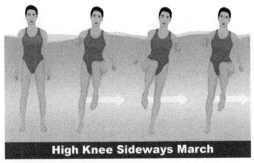

High Knee Sideways March

- Stand in chest high deep water
- March your left knee and swing your right arm at the same time
- Repeat with opposite side of body
- Move laterally through the pool, walking sideways, instead of front and back
- Continue for 30 seconds in one direction. Take a 15 second break, and repeat in reverse direction.
- Complete total of four sets

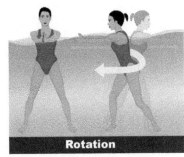

Rotation

- Stand with legs wide apart and arms extended with palms flat together
- Twist at your waist and drive your arms horizontally through water
- Rotate left and right at 180 degrees
- Complete four 30 second sets with 15 seconds rest in between

Figure Fifty

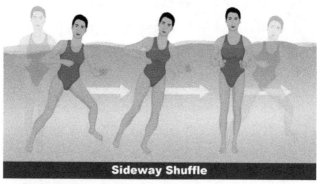

Sideway Shuffle

- Starting sideways lift your right leg and take a big step to the side
- Pull yourself sideways and bring legs together
- Begin a new set by switching directions
- Complete total of four sets, by resting for 15 seconds between sets.

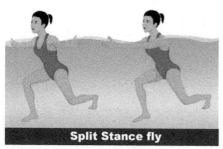

Split Stance fly

- Stand in the shallow part of the pool
- Keep hips square, step back with left leg and drop your left knee slightly
- Extend both arms to side, with palms facing forward
- Bring both arms together with palms touching and return arms to original position.
- Engage hips, legs and core
- This works your shoulders and upper back
- Complete four 30 second sets
- Rest 15 seconds in between and switch legs

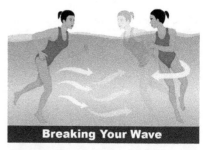

Breaking Your Wave

- Start in chest deep water and sprint down the length of the pool
- When you reach where you want to go, turn quickly and drive through the wake of water. This creates additional resistance
- Repeat for 5 minutes, resting in between sprints as needed.

How to Make Exercise Exciting Again?

How do you turn excuses into exciting reasons for you to start moving again? Here are some suggestions.

- **Try an out-of-the box exercise at least once a week**

One of the most common excuses for not exercising is boredom. Most people find "workout" synonymous with "work" which is something that is boring, taxing, and uninteresting. If you are doing the same gym routine everyday such as hitting the treadmill, stationary bike, free weights, or gym equipment –you can grow tired of this. An easy fix is to go out of your comfort zone and challenge yourself to try out a new exercise at least once a week. For example, if you're tired of yoga then try aerial yoga? There's drum fitness, Bollywood dancing, belly dancing, pole workouts, and hot yoga.

- **Invest in inexpensive, great looking workout clothes**

When you wear nice workout clothes instead of that old, flabby shirt, the chances are you get to feel more confident in yourself. Wearing fun colored gym leggings will also translate to a feeling of fun and activity.

Great, high quality gym gear can also affect your performance. A good sports bra or a high-quality pair of trendy sneakers will help you perform better in exercise. These will also give you better support from injury or pain.

- **Find a workout buddy**

When you have a workout buddy, you get to motivate each other, and you can give a certain level of commitment to turning up. You wouldn't want to lose a friend just because you're lazy or always late!

- **Get moving today!**

Nothing is a more perfect time to start than the present. The longer you delay, the harder it will be for you to get back into a good exercise routine. The key is to find activities that you enjoy so that working out will stop feeling like work for you.

Figure Fifty-One *(see next page)*

***

Lose-Your-Regain Activity # ten: Invite a Friend to Workout

Sticking to your exercise plans can be very challenging. You can boost motivation and accountability by asking a friend to join you.

Combine socializing with your daily movement and add fun to your exercise regime. Catch up with your friend while looking forward to your workout.

Exercise partners should be willing to make specific plans, and hold you accountable for it. Include specific goals like day, time, and duration for a timely and attainable behavior.

How to complete this skill:

- Approach a friend and ask if they would like to buddy up and get active at least a couple of days in the next seven days. Do research on exercise locations in your area that will work for a meet-up.

Have A Desk Job?

Use your work desk and chair to shape up

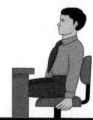

Pull Up

Work on arms and shoulders
- Sit upright
- Grasp sides of chair firmly with both hands
- Pull up firmly for a few seconds
- Let go

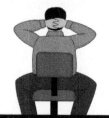

Neck muscle press

- Sit straight
- Clasp hands behind neck
- Hold elbows forward
- Pull forward with hands, pressing the head back at the same time

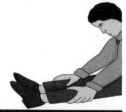

Tummy tightener

- Sit on clean floor with legs together and straight out
- Bend forward
- Grasp legs just below knees with hands
- At the same time, press up with legs

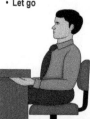

Arm Curl

Work on the upper arms
- Sit upright
- Grab the underside of your desk with palms upward
- Forearms should be parallel to desk
- Push up firmly for a few seconds
- Let go

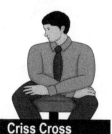

Criss Cross

Work on chest and legs
- Place feet 3-4 inches apart
- Bend forward and place hands on insides of opposite knees
- Press knees together
- At the same time hold them apart with both hands

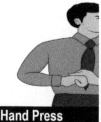

Hand Press

Work arms, chest and shoulders
- Sit upright in chair
- Hold arms across chest with one fist inside the other
- Press together firmly

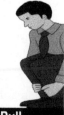

Back Pull

Work your back
- Keep your back straight
- Lean forward to comfortably grab your legs or knees
- Pull straight up using your back muscles

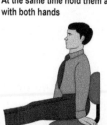

Leg lift

Work your shoulders, abdomen and arms
- Sit up straight on chair
- Lean forward and place palms against the side of the chair
- Hold legs straight out and hold for a few seconds
- Put feet back on floor

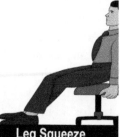

Leg Squeeze

Work on thighs, hips, calves and ankles
- Sit on forward edge of chair
- Lean back and hold legs straight
- Hook one foot over the other
- Hold tightly for a few seconds
- Rest feet on floor, keep legs straight
- Pull feet apart

- Decide on a plan for when, where, and how long you'll work out. Create a backup plan in case something does not go right, and try to figure out how you'll adapt.
- Try to be accountable to each other and commit to the time. Ask your friend to not let you bow out at the last minute.
- Have fun and get moving.

https://go.omadahealth.com (Health, Omada. "The Omada Program". n.d.)

***

Meet Tina, who has learned that eating is not just a social event, but that you can still eat healthy and enjoy food. She is now able to be a participant in her life and not just a bystander. She started a movement, a mindset and a motivation to reach the best phase of her life. Read about how she opened her mind to different people, approaches and ideas and found new solutions and resources for long-term success. Take a moment and explore your degree of open-mindedness

Figure Fifty-Two

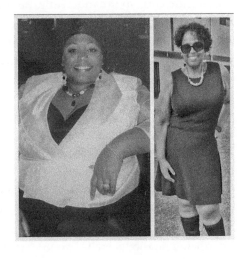

Tina: Battling to lose the weight I was carrying and to keep it off had been a challenge all my life. I tried every gimmick, pill, trick, and overnight remedy that I could find. Yo-Yo diets were true to their name; I was happy when I lost the weight and upset when I put the weight back on. Nothing worked! I began to feel lost and deserted. I was out of options; or so I told myself. Many people do not realize that before you conquer the physical aspect, you must first conquer the mind.

My weight loss battle went deeper than the physical realm. I struggled with secret behaviors that plagued my thoughts as well as my emotions. For a long time, I was a sneak eater. I would wait until I was alone and eat whatever I wanted and afterwards, I would hide the evidence. It was a mystery to my husband as to why I was gaining weight. I could fool him, but I was really fooling myself. If I couldn't get my mind under control, I would never get my weight under control. I had gotten to the point where my weight began to affect my health and the doctors were concerned about my heart. It was at this point that I began to reflect on my children. I couldn't bear to think about leaving them without their mother. In addition, my third daughter struggled with her weight. What example was I setting? If I could not defeat this giant, then, how could she? It was time to make an intentional decision about my life.

When my doctor told me that I needed to do something about my weight since he was unable to weigh me on his office scale anymore, it was the most embarrassing moment of my life. To add to it, my mother had a dream that my weight killed me and my children were grieving. I finally had weight loss surgery in 2015 and lost over 200 pounds. I decided to dedicate myself to my health.

After clearing the negative thoughts about weight loss being too hard, I could see that help had been in my view the entire time. That help was exercise. Initially, I had continually made the choice to reject exercise because I knew it would be work, work that I wasn't sure I could handle or wanted to handle. However, if I was going to succeed in losing weight, I needed to make a new choice. At first, I thought I had to choose differently if I wanted to see different results. During my fitness journey, I realized that it wasn't about getting different results. It was about my life. I had to choose differently to live differently. I understood the formula that if you do something consistently for thirty days you would create a new habit, if you continue to sixty days then you have created a new discipline but when you go past ninety days you have now created a new life style. It's a life style change, mentally, emotionally, and physically, that I was then and continue to be in pursuit of.

I spent so much time avoiding the very thing that is now my lifeline; exercise. I am going on four years of a daily exercise routine married to healthy nutritional eating habits which I document daily. My exercise regimen includes two to three hours a day of strength training, swimming, walking, and cardio. I joined MSTANY (Military Style Training Academy, New York) where I receive strength training and hi-intensity cardio; I swim two to three days each week, and walk a hiking trail. I also engage in a variety of activities on my own to keep my body moving such as, jumping rope, bike riding, kangaroo jumping, walking the beach, aerobics, trampoline, etc. I do these things by myself. I'm not looking for a partner or someone to tag along. I learned that I am responsible for myself. If my partner decided not to work out, I didn't want that to change my mind about working out. So, I go because it's me taking care of me. For me to be "FLY," (First love yourself), I must first love myself.

This is not an obsession; it's a mindset that broke the back of the couch potato. I just keep it moving. I work out six days a week, but I am mindful that balance is important. I give myself a day off to rest. I allow myself time, when I need it, without anxiety or remorse. I'm in command of my life and I changed the narrative of my life. It was an intentional decision that I must make every day; first in my mind, then my body follows. I have developed my own theme called #TinasTurn. This indicates that it's Tina's turn to take care of Tina. It's a movement, a mindset, and a motivation.

Chapter Eleven:

Glucose/Insulin Tolerance: The Carb Connection

"There are essential amino acids and essential fatty acids,
but there is no such thing as an essential carbohydrate."
– Richard K Bernstein, MD

*C*an I eat carbs after bariatric surgery?
How many carbs does my body need after surgery?
Do carbohydrates cause weight gain?
Carbohydrates often get a bad rap after bariatric surgery. Despite that, they are still a source of energy.

- Complex carbohydrates keep blood sugar levels stable and decrease carb cravings.
- Carbohydrates high in fiber fight constipation which is very common on a high protein diet.
- Eating the right amount of carbohydrates spares protein and prevents its conversion to fuel for the brain.

What's in Your Carb Wallet?

You know exactly how you feel when an intense craving for carbs strikes. Do you cave in or do you try your best to find a healthier substitute? So how exactly do you satisfy your carbohydrate fix?

Most cravings for carbs are believed to be derived from some sort of a physiological imbalance in your body. When cortisol, the stress hormone, goes up, it causes blood sugar levels to elevate as well. High levels of blood sugar release insulin, which is a fat- storing hormone that brings the sugar levels down but which also stores the sugar as fat. When you want to lose fat, you must take carbohydrates seriously.

When insulin overcompensates, it tricks your body into thinking it needs more energy and a vicious cycle starts. There is no universal way to eat carbohydrates because this will depend on what your individual goal is. It does not mean that all carbs are evil (Madsbad et al. 2014,70218-3).

Eat Carbs at the Right Time

I'm sure you've heard that it's best to eat carbs in the morning when you have the entire day to burn the carbohydrates you took in. But this habit may be something that will stop you from burning fat.

Remember that carbohydrates trigger the release of insulin, which is the hormone that encourages fat storage. When you are sleeping, your body is in an overnight fast so as you wake up, your insulin levels are low.

If you eat carbohydrates in the morning, you will suddenly have a major spike in insulin which will signal your body that it's got fuel. Instead of burning fat, it will go into fat storage mode. This energy spike can also lead to crashes making you hungry again by mid-morning, when you will more likely crave carbs again.

Another argument is that cortisol levels are at their peak in the morning. Cortisol is a stress hormone that rises throughout the night and reaches its peak in the morning as part of the body's natural wake - up cycle. The presence of cortisol in the morning can help facilitate weight loss, however, if combined with high levels of insulin, both can trigger the regeneration of fat cells.

It would be more beneficial to eat protein and healthy fats for breakfast and limit carbs for your evening meal. Eating carbs in the evening will limit these cortisol and insulin spikes. But take note that you cannot eat just any type of carbs!

Eat the Right Quality of Carbs

Not all carbs are created equal. Our enemies are the empty, processed carbs that are loaded with sugar and trigger fat storage. When your goal is to burn fat, you must eat quality carbohydrates.

But what, you might ask, are the right quality of carbs?

Good carbs are less- processed carbs that only have a mild impact on insulin and blood sugar. These include fruits and vegetables especially berries, apples, citrus, leafy greens, sweet potatoes, and squash.

Avoid the packaged and processed types like cakes, chips, cookies, and sugary treats. If it is made in a factory, then chances are that's a bad carb. Also avoid white rice, refined wheat flour, bread, and pasta.

Eat the Right Quantity of Carbs

Portion control is very important when it comes to carbs. Just because you are eating at the right time and in the right quantity does not give you the license to consume a massive bowl of fruit. Instead of calorie counting, the best way is to limit your portions. A three to four ounce. portion is usually sufficient to satisfy your hunger.

You can also use your hand as a guide. If you are eating more than a palm- full, then you already need to limit your food. This will stop you from overeating and not to eat when you're already full.

Eat Carbs with Other Healthy Food

When eating carbs, it is best to eat them with protein or healthy fat. This will help you achieve optimum fat loss versus eating carbs alone.
This is because eating protein and healthy fat with carbs will slow down the digestive process, slowing the release of sugar into the blood stream. This means it requires less of an insulin response. This means you can still enjoy carbs while in fat- burning mode, as your insulin is not yet announcing that you are already in storage mode. Choose lean protein and healthy fats to eat with carbs. Of course, portion control is still recommended.

Lowering Your Carb Intake

In an ideal world, you would be consuming thirty grams of carbs a day. At this number, the fat practically melts off. When you have been eating hundreds of grams of carbs all your life, it gets to be practically impossible to reach the ideal number. The goal is to start off at a manageable number like eighty grams and keep lowering your carb intake until you can get as close to forty grams as possible.

Figure Fifty-Three

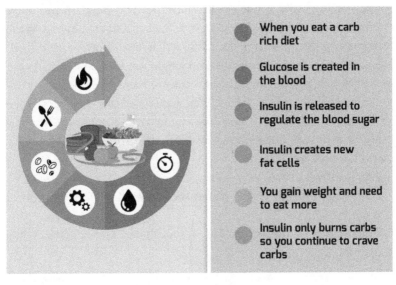

When you eat a carb rich diet

Glucose is created in the blood

Insulin is released to regulate the blood sugar

Insulin creates new fat cells

You gain weight and need to eat more

Insulin only burns carbs so you continue to crave carbs

If salty carbs like potato chips and pretzels are your thing, then opt for something similar in texture such as:

- Roasted chickpeas.
- Baked parmesan crisps.
- Raw carrots and hummus.
- Cucumber slices and tuna salad.

If sweet carbs like chocolate and candy are your fixations, opt for quick and easy choices like:

- Small banana with almond butter.
- Frozen or fresh berries with low fat cottage cheese.
- Chocolate protein shake.
- Small square of 80% dark chocolate.

If starchy carbs are on your mind, in addition to your protein meal and veggies, opt for:

- Cauliflower substitutes (rice, mashed and pizza crust).
- Spaghetti squash or zucchini noodles.
- Quinoa.
- Almond butter banana muffins.
- Homemade granola: (chopped almonds, uncooked rolled oats, scoop of vanilla /chocolate protein powder, coconut flakes, sunflower seeds, and unsweetened freeze-dried fruit).

***

Carb Cycling and Weight Loss Surgery

Carb cycling is like calorie cycling discussed in *Chapter three*, but over here, the amount of carbs will be varied instead of the entire caloric intake.

Carb cycling was originally a program developed for bodybuilders, but can work to jumpstart the weight loss after bariatric surgery. The key is not to be good on a low carb day and go crazy on the other days. Successful weight loss involves eating good quality carbs with adequate protein. Best results with weight loss are seen if you allocate one or two days a week to high carb days. If you decide on more than one day a week, make sure they are never back to back. Carb cycling is designed only for short-term use.

Carb cycling involves more time and energy than a low carb diet. If you are having success with your current low-carb diet, then stick to it. Do not fix something that is not broken.

Carb cycling involves:

- **Knowing yourself:** If you cannot stick to portion sizes, then carb cycling is not for you.
- **Planning:** If you dislike tracing your meals or prepping, carb cycling is not for you.

- **Picking wisely:** High carb days consist of fruit, non-starchy vegetables, and complex carbohydrates. It is not a license to eat cookies and cupcakes.
- **Be ready to return:** If you see your weight stalling with two days of carb cycling, return to a low carb diet.

Sample Carb Cycling plan: Here is an example of how to do the five-day carb cycling plan, using eighty grams of carbs as the highest amount on a high day:

- **Day one**: Eighty grams of carbs.
- **Day two**: Fifty grams of carbs.
- **Day three**: Forty grams of carbs.
- **Day four**: Fifty grams of carbs.
- **Day five**: Eighty grams of carbs.

***

You had weight loss surgery but still struggle with a sugar addiction. Staying on a low-carb diet after surgery must include restriction of sugar. View sugar addiction as an allergy,if you want to be in total control. Old habits lead you to desire sweets even though the consequences are not good. The first bite of sugar sends a dopamine rush to the brain, which makes you feel happy.

Kicking the Sugar Habit

In my experience of guiding bariatric patients who have sugar cravings, I see that it is not enough to merely cut back on sugar, but to eliminate it for a certain period. A three-day sugar fix is when you can go three days without any sugar (even sugar substitutes). After your palate starts readjusting without any sugar during the three-day period, even an apple will taste extremely sweet. You will start becoming more aware of the natural sweetness in milk. Withdrawal symptoms may include headaches, fatigue, and irritability but the positive affects you feel afterward are worth the three days of abstinence.

CAUTION: Please consult your physician if you suffer from hypoglycemia, insulin resistance, and diabetes. Also, if you are on insulin or oral medications to control blood sugar please do not attempt this.

During the three days:

- No food or drinks with added sugar. This includes even the sugar you add to your morning coffee.
- No artificial sweeteners.
- No fruit.
- No dairy.
- No starches like bread, potatoes, and rice.

- Increase protein intake.
- Stick with vegetables.
- Stay full eating nuts as snacks.
- Hydrate well.
- No alcohol.

Figure Fifty-Four

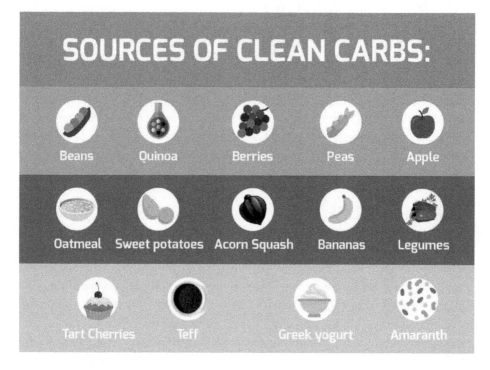

Some sources of Clean Carbs:
- Beans
- Quinoa
- Berries
- Peas
- Apples
- Oatmeal
- Sweet potatoes
- Acorn squash
- Legumes
- Tart Cherries
- Teff (nutty grain like quinoa)

- Greek yogurt
- Amaranth (gluten free complete protein grain)

***

Sweet Confusion: Taming Your Sweet Tooth

As a bariatric patient, perpetuating an unhealthy addiction to sweets creates havoc with the weight loss process

Treat them equally: As per David Katz, MD, founding director of the Yale-Griffin Prevention Research Center, taste buds are unable to distinguish between raw sugar and high fructose corn syrup (Katz,2017).

Do the math: Four grams of sugar equals one teaspoon of sugar. When reading food labels divide the number of grams of sugar by four.

Falling for the fake: Artificial sweeteners are non-caloric chemicals that stimulate the sweet receptors in the mouth. These chemicals are 600 times sweeter than sugar and cultivate a preference for more sugar.

Curb Omega- 6 fatty acids: Sugar in your diet activates the conversion of omega - 6 fatty acids found in vegetable oils into arachidonic acid, and generates inflammation, as per Barry Sears, creator of the Zone diet. He believes that an omega - 6 fatty rich diet along with refined carbs is a recipe for disaster (Sears,1999).

Fruit over fruit juice: As per Henry S. Lodge, MD, co-author of the bestselling book *Younger Next year: Live Strong, Fit and Sexy- Until You're 80 and Beyond,* while an orange contributes four teaspoons of sugar that is absorbed by the body over a few hours, eight ounces of orange juice contains eight teaspoons of sugar absorbed by the body in twenty minutes. (Crowley and Lodge,2007).

Low sugar fruit: Prioritize fruit like raspberries, strawberries and clementine's (fruits that take longer to break down) over a banana, which converts to sugar quickly.

Figure Fifty-Five *(see next page)*

***

Resistant Starches

Resistant starches are those that pass through your large bowel and stay undigested. They help with fermentation and produce short chain fatty acids and ketones for your gut friendly bugs (Gundry, 2017).

You want to be getting more of the following in your bariatric diet:

- Parsnips
- Turnips
- Jicama
- Jerusalem artichokes

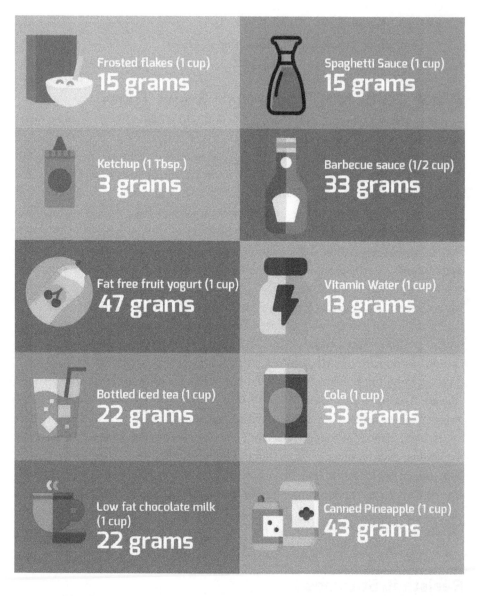

Frosted flakes (1 cup)
15 grams

Spaghetti Sauce (1 cup)
15 grams

Ketchup (1 Tbsp.)
3 grams

Barbecue sauce (1/2 cup)
33 grams

Fat free fruit yogurt (1 cup)
47 grams

Vitamin Water (1 cup)
13 grams

Bottled iced tea (1 cup)
22 grams

Cola (1 cup)
33 grams

Low fat chocolate milk (1 cup)
22 grams

Canned Pineapple (1 cup)
43 grams

- Taro root
- Shirataki noodles
- Unripe papaya
- Unripe mango

These resistant starches increase satiety, improve your sensitivity to insulin and cut down fat storage.

***

Carbohydrate Swapping

After bariatric surgery, high carbohydrate foods lead to weight regain. If before surgery, pizza, cereal, and potatoes were the cornerstone of your diet, cutting back is a struggle after bariatric surgery. To maintain the weight you have already lost, start experimenting with lower carb options. Each carb rich food has three or more swaps that might work for you as you join the losers club.

Figure Fifty-Six

HIGH CARB FOODS	HEALTHIER SWAPS
PIZZA/NOODLES	ZUCCHINI NOODLES SPAGHETTI SQUASH
SANDWICH BREAD	LETTUCE WRAPS
PIZZA CRUST	CAULIFLOWER PIZZA CRUST
POTATO CHIPS	PARMESAN CRISPS
FRENCH FRIES	GREEN BEAN FRIES, CARROT FRIES, SWEET POTATO FRIES
MASHED POTATOES	MASHED CAULIFLOWER
BREAKFAST CEREAL	OLD FASHIONED OATS UNSWEETENED YOGURT
BREADCRUMBS	CRUSHED NUTS
RICE	QUINOA CAULIFLOWER RICE
CRACKERS	CUCUMBER SLICES

***

Figure Fifty-Seven

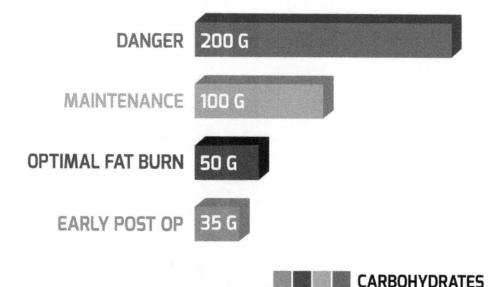

BARIATRIC CARB ZONES

DANGER — 200 G
MAINTENANCE — 100 G
OPTIMAL FAT BURN — 50 G
EARLY POST OP — 35 G

CARBOHYDRATES

Ref: http://www.bariatriceating.com/
Early post op phase: Thirty five grams of carbohydrates
Optimal fat burn phase: Fifty grams of carbohydrates
Maintenance phase: Hundred grams of carbohydrates
Danger phase: Two hundred grams of carbohydrates

The website http://www.*bariatriceating.com/* has a well- explained info-graphic which breaks down the various carb zones throughout your bariatric journey. Based on that information the various bariatric carb zones are discussed further below.

Early Post op phase (< thirty-five grams): You just had bariatric surgery and are dropping weight. You can hardly eat your calories during the early post-op period.

During the **Optimal Fat Loss phase** (thirty-five to fifty grams), you are getting your carbs from veggies, yogurt, and lower carb fruit.

During the **Maintenance phase** (seventy-five to hundred grams) you are eating mostly good carbs like sweet potatoes, beans, and fruit but in larger portions.

During the **Danger phase** (hundred to two hundred grams), you have gone back to your bad habits of eating processed and convenience foods like bread, pasta, rice, crackers, sugar, soda, chips, and cereal. You have regained most or even all your weight back.

***

What is Bariatric keto?

You hear about it everywhere.

Can I go on a keto diet after bariatric surgery?

I am losing a lot of weight on the keto diet?

Does the keto diet meet bariatric protocols?

Losing weight on the keto diet is not the issue, it is keeping the weight off that is the problem. In the past, you have been on an innumerable number of diets to lose weight. Once you get off the diet, you see yourself gaining the weight back.

Mainstream keto is not the suitable mindset for bariatric patients. The protein, fat and caloric needs are very different due to the reduced capacity of the stomach pouch and its absorption capabilities.

Keto diets should also be avoided by diabetic's, patients with gallbladder and liver issues and women who are breast feeding (Paoli, 2014,2092-2107).

A mainstream keto diet consists of a high fat-moderate protein-low carb diet.

- The high fat diet leads to low glucose levels.
- The body releases stored triglycerides.
- Fatty acids move to the liver.
- The liver produces ketones.

A Bariatric keto diet would consist of **Low carb-moderate fat-high protein diet**

Figure Fifty-Eight *(see next page)*

- Stay between thirty grams of carbs a day and not more than forty grams' net carbs a day.
- Do not restrict fiber intake.
- Keep lean protein around hundred grams a day.
- Stay satisfied with fat intake.
- Limit your snacks.
- Hydrate well.

How is the traditional keto diet different from the bariatric keto diet?

EAT	AVOID
CHICKEN.	HEAVY CREAM
TURKEY	CREAM CHEESE
FISH	UNLIMITED BACON
SEAFOOD	OATS
EGGS	QUINOA
BEEF	BARLEY
PORK	WHEAT MORE THAN 1 TSP OF BUTTER
OLIVE OIL	ALCOHOL.
COCONUT OIL	BEANS AND LEGUMES
AVOCADO OIL	STARCHY VEGETABLES
PLAIN GREEK YOGURT	FRUITS HIGH IN CARBS LIKE GRAPES,
HARD CHEESE	MANGO ORANGES, PAPAYA, BANANA AND DRIED FRUIT
COTTAGE CHEESE	CHOCOLATE
ALMONDS	MILK
MACADAMIA NUTS	HONEY/MAPLE SYRUP
NUT BUTTER	COOKIES
TOMATOES	CHIPS
EGGPLANT	CANDY
BROCCOLI	POTATOES
AVOCADO	RICE
GREEN BEANS	PASTA
CABBAGE	

Figure Fifty-Nine: Traditional Keto Diet *(see next page)*

Keep in mind:

- As per bariatric recommendations, a bariatric post op patient needs at least sixty to a hundred grams of protein a day

Macronutrient Ratios	• 70% fats • 25% protein • 5% carbohydrates
On 1000 calories a day, the macro breakdown is:	**FAT** 70% fat 700 calories from fat 78 grams of fat
	PROTEIN 25% protein 250 calories from protein 62.5 grams of protein
	CARBOHYDRATES 5% carbohydrates 50 calories from carbohydrates 12.5 grams of carbohydrates

- Tolerating high levels of fat is tough for some bariatric patients
- Food intolerances after bariatric surgery create less variety in meals

Figure Sixty: Bariatric Keto Diet

Macronutrient Ratios	• 40% fats • 45% protein • 15% carbohydrates
On 1000 calories a day the macro breakdown	**FAT** 40% fat 400 calories from fat 44.4 grams of fat
	PROTEIN 45% protein 450 calories from protein 112.5 grams of protein
	CARBOHYDRATES 15% carbohydrates 150 calories from carbohydrates 37.5 grams of carbohydrates

Figure Sixty-One

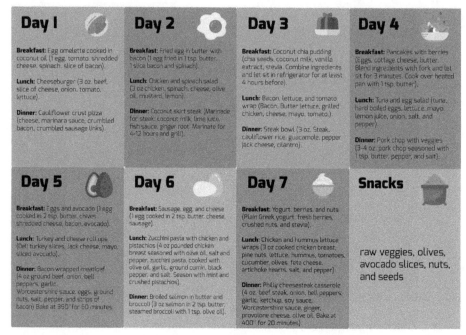

| **Day 1** | **Day 2** | **Day 3** | **Day 4** |

Day 1

Breakfast: Egg omelette cooked in coconut oil (1 egg, tomato, shredded cheese, spinach, slice of bacon).

Lunch: Cheeseburger (3 oz. beef, slice of cheese, onion, tomato, lettuce).

Dinner: Cauliflower crust pizza (cheese, marinara sauce, crumbled bacon, crumbled sausage links).

Day 2

Breakfast: Fried egg in butter with bacon (1 egg fried in 1 tsp. butter, 1 slice bacon and spinach).

Lunch: Chicken and spinach salad (3 oz chicken, spinach, cheese, olive oil, mustard, lemon).

Dinner: Coconut skirt steak (Marinade for steak: coconut milk, lime juice, fish sauce, ginger root. Marinate for 4-12 hours and grill).

Day 3

Breakfast: Coconut chia pudding (chia seeds, coconut milk, vanilla extract, stevia. Combine ingredients and let sit in refrigerator for at least 4 hours before).

Lunch: Bacon, lettuce, and tomato wrap (Bacon, Butter lettuce, grilled chicken, cheese, mayo, tomato.).

Dinner: Steak bowl (3 oz. Steak, cauliflower rice, guacamole, pepper jack cheese, cilantro).

Day 4

Breakfast: Pancakes with berries (Eggs, cottage cheese, butter. Blend ingredients with fork and let sit for 3 minutes. Cook over heated pan with 1 tsp. butter).

Lunch: Tuna and egg salad (tuna, hard boiled eggs, lettuce, mayo, lemon juice, onion, salt, and pepper).

Dinner: Pork chop with veggies (3-4 oz. pork chop seasoned with 1 tsp. butter, pepper, and salt).

Day 5

Breakfast: Eggs and avocado (1 egg cooked in 2 tsp. butter, chives, shredded cheese, bacon, avocado).

Lunch: Turkey and cheese roll ups (Deli turkey slices, Jack cheese, mayo, sliced avocado).

Dinner: Bacon wrapped meatloaf (4 oz ground beef, onion, bell peppers, garlic, Worcestershire sauce, eggs, ground nuts, salt, pepper, and strips of bacon) Bake at 350° for 60 minutes.

Day 6

Breakfast: Sausage, egg, and cheese (1 egg cooked in 2 tsp. butter, cheese, sausage).

Lunch: Zucchini pasta with chicken and pistachios (4 oz pounded chicken breast seasoned with olive oil, salt and pepper, zucchini pasta, cooked with olive oil, garlic, ground cumin, black pepper, and salt. Season with mint and crushed pistachios).

Dinner: Broiled salmon in butter and broccoli (3 oz salmon in 2 tsp. butter, steamed broccoli with 1 tsp. olive oil).

Day 7

Breakfast: Yogurt, berries, and nuts (Plain Greek yogurt, fresh berries, crushed nuts, and stevia).

Lunch: Chicken and hummus lettuce wraps (3 oz cooked chicken breast, pine nuts, lettuce, hummus, tomatoes, cucumber, olives, feta cheese, artichoke hearts, salt, and pepper).

Dinner: Philly cheesesteak casserole (4 oz. beef steak, onion, bell peppers, garlic, ketchup, soy sauce, Worcestershire sauce, ginger, provolone cheese, olive oil. Bake at 400° for 20 minutes).

Snacks

raw veggies, olives, avocado slices, nuts, and seeds

***

Lose-Your-Regain Activity # eleven: Gradual change

Quick fixes are tempting, but they don't build the skills we need to handle setbacks. Challenging ourselves one step at a time and avoiding deprivation leads to the best results.

At every step in the process, consider what works or does not work and adjust your plans as needed. Remember perfection is not your goal. You don't need to make the best possible choice every time, just a better one as often as possible.

- Pick a goal you feel is doable and measurable.
- Set a time frame to accomplish it.
- Focus on a behavior you have complete control over (e.g. behaviors like not skipping lunch, rather than outcomes like weight loss).

Answer the following questions:

1. What specific goal would you like to reach?
2. What daily action do you need to accomplish that will bring you closer to that goal?
3. How do you plan to track your daily action?
4. How do you plan on rewarding yourself without food if you stick to the plan?

5.   Are you willing to commit to taking action every day? Why or why not?
https://go.omadahealth.com
(Health, Omada. "The Omada Program". n.d)

***

Meet Karen who believes bariatric surgery changed her life, with a newfound outlook for the future. She has all this positive energy that she can apply toward herself and her family. Read about how she defines her life through her choices. Today, work on accepting your life and begin to live it fully here and now.

Figure Sixty-Two

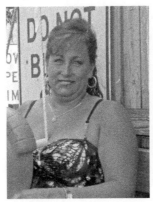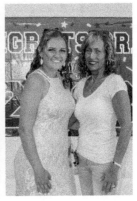

Karen: My weight loss journey began almost two years before the actual surgical procedure. Battling obesity was discouraging and exhausting. No matter what diet, weight loss program or exercise regimen I attempted it was always two steps forward three steps back. My health began to decline.

Being obese was painful, not only physically, but emotionally as well. I knew I had to do something to prevent the inevitable. I began researching and educating myself on the different surgical procedures available, planning financially and mentally, and preparing myself for what, unknown to me, would prove to be one of the most pivotal decisions I would make. With the guidance of my outstanding surgical team, I decided the procedure would be the Roux-n-y gastric bypass.

My surgery date was December 12, 2013. The day of my surgery I was 225 pounds. and my BMI was thirty eight. During just one year, I lost 115 pounds. and my BMI sank to twenty-three. In addition, within three months my health was greatly improving. No more sleep apnea, my cholesterol and blood sugar levels were within normal range, acid reflux had completely disappeared.

Fast forward to the present year 2018. I celebrate five years of maintaining my weight loss goal. I attribute my success to my understanding that weight loss surgery is not a cure for obesity but rather a tool that I use to fight my battle. If I were to rely solely on the bypass surgery I would surely fail. I keep my before-surgery pictures close by as a visual reminder of the agony of obesity. I changed my relationship with food. Although I do take supplements, nutrition is my focus. For me following the basic rules makes maintaining my weight easy. Three meals a day. No grazing or snacking.

I choose low fat, high protein, and sugar free foods. I sit down to enjoy my meals and I still chew, chew, and chew! I drink plenty of water and stay away from alcohol. I no longer turn to food for comfort, instead, I turn to activity and exercise to vent my frustrations.

My surgery has not limited me in any way. I still enjoy dining out. Most importantly, I made a commitment to myself. I did not put myself through a barrage of diagnostic tests and major surgery only to find myself right back where I started.

Chapter Twelve:
Acceptance to Portion Control

"The surest way to make your dreams come true is to live them."
– Roy T. Bennett

A s you eat, your stomach (along with other fatty tissues) secretes leptin, which sends a signal to your brain that you are full. The problem is you don't always listen to it, especially when you are eating a meal of fat, sugar, or salt. The reward circuits in your brain light up and override the body's response to leptin. This leads to an urge to eat the entire stack of cookies.

Putting your fork or the cookie down between bites helps to tap the brakes, giving your brain a chance to catch up and realize the "I'm full" message being pumped out by your digestive hormones.

Figure Sixty-Three

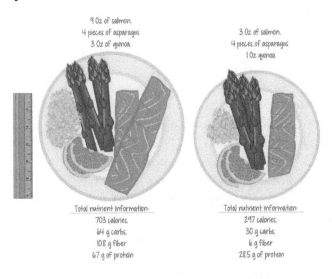

9 Oz of salmon.
4 pieces of asparagus
3 Oz of quinoa

3 Oz of salmon.
4 pieces of asparagus
1 Oz quinoa

Total nutrient information:
703 calories.
64 g carbs.
108 g fiber
67 g of protein

Total nutrient information:
297 calories.
30 g carbs.
6 g fiber
28.5 g of protein

Avoiding portion distortion is crucial to weight control. Pay attention to the size of your portions since just an extra 100-200 calories a day can add to your weight gain. Though WHAT you eat is incredibly important as a bariatric patient, HOW MUCH you eat is also largely responsible for weight changes.

Mastering the Hunger Quotient

Overeating is probably one of the primary reasons why people gain weight and become obese. The saying that "too much of anything is bad for you" is applicable when it comes to food because too much food equals calories, and unburned calories leads to extra pounds.

The conveniences of the modern world make it easy for us to overeat.

There are just too many chances nowadays to overeat. Unlike ancient humans who had to hunt for and gather for food, now you can just click an app and food comes to you. You don't even need to speak to anyone to get your meal.

Not to mention supermarkets at every corner, restaurants, food bazaars, and all-you-can-eat buffets that are just too tempting to ignore, even if you are not hungry. How many times have you reached for that chocolate chip cookie "just because," or had an ice cream on a whim?

But do we just need to eat when we're just hungry? Is this the key to losing weight?

The Hunger Quotient

I encountered the concept of the hunger quotient from the website https://nutritiouslife.com/ and according to this website the key to controlling the portions of what we eat is to listen to our body and master our hunger quotient. Use it as a tool to keep you on track.

Figure Sixty-Four *(see next page)*

Hunger/Fullness Quotients

1. **Stuffed** (like you want to unbutton your pants at the table): I am never going to eat again.
2. **Extremely full**: I couldn't eat another bite.
3. **Satisfied**: I could have skipped those last few bites.
4. **Slightly satisfied/just right**: I feel satisfied with not one bit of fullness.
5. **Neutral**: I'm not hungry or full.
6. **Slightly hungry**: I guess I'm about ready to eat.
7. **Hungry**: I'm ready for another meal.
8. **Very hungry**: I'm ready for a big meal.

HUNGER 1-10	FOOD, AMOUNT AND TIME	FULLNESS	FEELINGS/ MOOD
	BREAKFAST/TIME		
	MORNING SNACK/TIME		
	LUNCH/TIME		
	AFTERNOON SNACK/TIME		

9. **Extremely hungry**: I can't even check my social media feed until I eat something.
10. **Famished (Ready to pass out)**: Don't talk to me until I eat-I may eat my shirt.

https://nutritiouslife.com/

What exactly is the hunger quotient? The hunger quotient measures your level of hunger with "one" being extremely full and "ten" being extremely starving.

It is interesting to see the levels because it explains a person's stages of being hungry and suggests that to avoid overeating, you must always be between stage "four" and "six", between being "slightly satisfied" and "slightly hungry".

I do agree that following this has its merits because if you don't wait for your body to feel starved, then you would not need to eat everything that's within your reach. When you feel famished, of course a small plateful of food will never be enough. You would have to get a second, third, and even fourth serving to satisfy your hunger.

However, if you eat when you're slightly hungry and stop when you feel slightly satiated, then overeating may be avoided. https://nutritiouslife.com/

How to Know When to Stop?

Mastering the hunger quotient is not a very easy thing to do because when we're hungry the tendency is for us to eat quickly. Before even realizing that we're already full, we have already eaten more than what we should have eaten.

New alarms start setting off in the post-bariatric surgery body, as a warning system that you are getting close to feeling full. While some hiccup, others sneeze or have a runny nose. The vagus nerve regulates various aspects of the body along with digestion. This sensor that runs from the brain to our gut stimulates these 'almost there" responses. Not everyone experiences this, but if you do, then it's a signal to stop eating.

Embrace an environment that supports your intention of a successful life after bariatric surgery. You have the choice of either adjusting to the new norm or feeling like you are constantly depriving yourself and being on an endless diet. Changing your living space around for convenience and easy access helps in supporting one's goals. Setting up your kitchen with smaller dishes and bowls on the lower shelves along with setting up a cabinet with reusable containers for leftovers works well.

In addition to eating smaller portions it is imperative the food tastes good. This prevents feelings of restriction or regret. A supportive environment helps you focus on other aspects of being successful after bariatric surgery.

***

Calorie density is an important concept when there are issues with portion control. Caloric density can be determined by dividing the number of calories per serving by the number of grams per serving.

Calorie Density or Volumetrics

Calorie density refers to the calories per bite of food and can be easily lowered without altering the palatability of food. Calories in every bite can be cut by changing the amount of water in foods. While this adds weight and volume, it does not add calories. You can lower the caloric density of a casserole by adding more vegetables, which have a high content of water.

Larger portion sizes lead to huge increases in calories a day, which can easily go unnoticed. As per Barbara Rolls, MD, Chair of Nutritional Sciences at Penn

State University, even though we might eat the same volume of food every day, just being exposed to larger portions seems to override this tendency, leading us to more intake. Lowering the caloric density of these big portions might still thwart weight gain, compared to calorie dense portions (Rolls,2007).

Calories can be cut by reducing the fat, and adding vegetables and fruit to the bariatric diet. Low-fat brownies, baked potato chips might be low in fat but they are not low on the calorie density scale. In published studies by Barbara Rolls, MD caloric density was changed by adding vegetables to breakfast, lunch, and dinner (Rolls,2007).

Caloric density is calculated by dividing the calories by the weight in grams. While higher density foods may be worse, portion size is what ultimately matters. Check out the caloric density of a traditional meal of General Tso's chicken below. Adding vegetables and making some healthier switches, results in a larger volumetric meal with lower calories.

Figure Sixty-Five

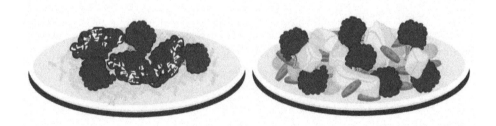

TRADITIONAL MEAL	HOW WE CUT THE CALORIE DENSITY	VOLUMETRICS
General Tsao's Chicken with sticky sauce, cauliflower rice and broccoli	* Add more vegetables * Reduce fat and sugar in sauce * Switch from fried, skin-on chicken to chicken breast fillet * Switch to quinoa or cauliflower rice	Chicken-Broccoli Stir-Fry with Water Chestnuts and Carrots

Portion Size Mistakes You Might Be Making

Chances are you might be eating too much of a certain food. Remember over-indulging in high protein foods can also derail your weight loss, if you eat too much of them.

- **High protein cereal**

When was the last time you measured your high protein cereal before preparing your breakfast? Do you check the nutrition facts label to determine the correct serving sizes? For some high protein cereals, one cup is the recommended serving size. This would not work as a bariatric serving size. Chances are you are eating more than what is recommended by your dietitian.

- **Chicken breast**

You have been told that lean protein is healthy, right? Not if you are eating too much of it. Eating an entire chicken breast is way above the bariatric portion size. The recommended portion is three to four ounces of chicken. Depending on the vendor, some chicken breasts are two to three times the size of what you need. Extra calories from chicken can add up and ruin your progress.

- **Fruit**

A healthy serving of fruit is a great alternative to a sugary high fat dessert. You still need to watch your caloric and carb intake with fruit. When adding fruit to smoothies it is imperative to stick to portion sizes. Consider the sugar and carbohydrate content of fruit. Stay away from dried fruit like dried cranberries, apricots, or raisins due to higher sugar content. Get out your calculator before you start chomping on fruit.

- **Salad dressing:**

Though salads are encouraged, it is the salad dressing that can add calories. Some restaurant salads contain over 500 calories in fatty dressing. Salad calories vary greatly but a few numbers to give you an idea when eating out:

  - Grilled chicken Caesar salad: 770 calories.
  - Cobb salad: 1130 calories.
  - Greek salad: 500 calories.
  - Taco salad: 830 calories.
  - Oriental crispy chicken salad: 1450 calories.

The dressing and ingredients you choose along with portion sizes will change your salad calories. Avoid the following unhealthy salad ingredients that fill your plate with needless fat and useless calories:

  - Bacon.
  - Croutons.
  - Creamy dressings.
  - Processed deli meats.
  - Crispy, battered, breaded foods.
  - Wontons.
  - Honey glazed food items.
  - Taco bowl.

- **Cooking spray:**

You skip the oil and butter to cook healthier meals at home. You use a cooking spray to avoid calories, but may be neglecting to account for calories from the cooking spray. A single serving of spray is quarter of a second. The center for Science in Public Interest did an evaluation on cooking sprays and came up with the information that a typical six- second spray contributed fifty calories and six grams of fat.

- **Coffee creamer:**

Your morning cup of coffee might be the most fattening and unhealthy thing you consume depending on the serving size of your creamer. A single serving of liquid creamer is one tablespoon. The small amount of fat in each serving adds up, depending on how many cups of coffee you drink all day.

These measuring tricks will help your control your portions:

Figure Sixty-Six *(see next page)*

***

Mind Over Meal

While measuring serving sizes works for some people, other do not have the patience to measure their food. Whether it's a psychological reason or they just find it tiresome, it's a technique that might not be for everyone.

So, what can you do if you have the same problem? How can you control your portions? You might be surprised but there are people who reported that by changing the way they eat, they are able to eat less and manage their serving sizes. Here are some options that you can try out.

Eat slowly.

This is what is called mindful eating. Chew your food slowly, eat in small bites and appreciate every flavor of the food you're eating. This way your body can slowly adjust to your food intake which can help you identify if you are already full.

Eat every few hours.

If you have an overeating problem, one good way is to try scheduling a small snack every three to four hours.

Eat nutritionally dense foods.

Foods high in nutrients are more filling than those with empty calories, like sugar-rich foods. When eating a meal try to eat protein or vegetables first, instead of the carbs on your plate.

BASEBALL

1 cup of starch (oatmeal, sweet potato).

DECK OF CARDS

3-4 ounces of poultry or meat.

CHECKBOOK

4 ounces of fish.

SHOT GLASS

2 tablespoons oil or salad dressing.

PACKAGE OF DENTAL FLOSS

1 ounce of a treat: a cookie or piece of chocolate.

A LIP STICK CAP

1 teaspoon of peanut butter.

2 PING PONG BALLS

1 ounce of nuts.

1 GOLF BALL

2 Tablespoons of peanut butter.

A PAIR OF DICE

1 ounce of cheese.

A HALF DOLLAR

1 teaspoon of salad dressing.

SIZE OF A POSTAGE STAMP

1 teaspoon of margarine or butter.

Count your condiments.

A little ketchup or a little extra hummus does matter. Measure them out just like anything else. A heaping spoon of peanut butter may end up being two tablespoons rather than one, thereby doubling your caloric intake from ninety-five calories to 199 calories.

Mix and match your menu.

Eat a variety of healthy foods that can promote the feeling of fullness instead of empty calories. Examples of these are protein, fiber-rich foods and heart-healthy fats. Eating a different combination with different flavors and textures also helps you satisfy your palate, because of the appetizing mix.

Blue Plate Special

As per Brian Wansink, Ph.D, director of the Cornell University Food and Brand Lab, a plate's specific color does not cause you to overeat. It all happens when the color of your plate contrasts with the color of the food you eat. White rice served on a white plate leads to a 30% increase in intake, more than if the plate were blue in color. (http://www.mindlesseating.org/pdf/Mindless_Dieting_01.pdf)

Dish Deception

A study by Cornell University Researchers found that when people were given a larger bowl, they served themselves 3% more without even noticing. A large serving spoon also increased their serving by 14.5%. The alarming thing was that the study used nutrition experts as their subjects, so imagine how it would be for the regular person. So, when you are trying to control your portions, especially if you're indulging in a dessert, use a small platter and a teaspoon. When baking, use mini muffin cups and smaller baking trays. Use a standard recipe and just make smaller portions. Fool your brain into thinking you are eating more.

Utensil Selection

Cut calories by using tongs instead of serving spoons to serve food. It is harder to grab food with tongs and you end up serving less. The smallest details, like forks, knives, and spoons, affect our portion sizes.

As humans, we develop expectations for how food tastes based on past eating experiences. Defying these assumptions and introducing unusual variations in cutlery increases the satisfaction of the snack or meal. New ingredients, new flavors, new plates, and different cutlery help you refocus on what you are eating.

Serving Style

In one of Wansink's studies, he found that people ate 25-30% less when food was served from the stove top, than when served family style at the table. Just getting up to go serve yourself more food deters you from doing it (Wansink & Sobol,2007,106-123).

Low Beams

As per Wansink, while bright lighting prods you to eat faster and eat more, dim lighting creates a calming environment, encourages you to pay attention to your food and helps you avoid overeating (Wansink & Sobol,2007,106-123).

Portion Control Containers

A great tool in taking the guesswork out of portion sizes is to use the various portion control containers out there in the market. They eliminate the chore of weighing your food and staying in control of how much to eat.

Use Ziplocs or containers to portion your food.

If you are cooking a big batch of food, divide it by using Ziplocs or containers that you can easily store in the fridge and reheat. This technique works for raw food as well as cooked food.

Use mason jars to pack salads.

The tricky part of packing your own salads to take to work is how to make sure that your salad will not turn soggy by lunch time. The answer to this problem is the amazing mason jar!
When building your salad, place the dressing first at the bottom of the jar then place the heavier, meaty ingredients next such as tomatoes, tofu, onions, and cucumber. The lighter the vegetable, the last it should be in the order which means your salad greens should be last in line. This technique will keep the greens crisp rather than soggy because they are not weighed down by the heavier veggies which are at the bottom of the jar. When it's time for lunch, you can easily shake the jar to distribute the dressing evenly.

The Left-Overs- First Policy When Ordering Out

When you find, yourself eating out, a great trick is to immediately ask your server to bag a portion or at least half of your meal. This means you are not tempted to finish the entire plate.

***

Figure Sixty-Seven *(see next page)*

Knives Over Forks: The Art of Taking Tiny Bites

Have you ever opened the freezer, taken out a gallon of ice cream, and used a tiny spoon to scoop through the frozen goodness?

WHICH IS MORE FILLING?

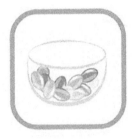 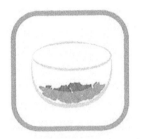 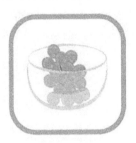

Jelly Beans   **Chocolate Chips**   **Grapes**

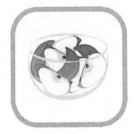 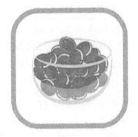

Apples   **Cherry Tomatoes**

As per Barbara Rolls, professor at the Helen Guthrie chair of nutritional Sciences at Penn State and past-president of The Obesity Socienty and the society for the study of ingestive behaviour, each of these snacks contribute 100 calories.

But after eating a calorie-dense food like jelly beans, you're less likely to feel full and more likely to keep eating. When researchers lower calorie density by 25 percent. people eat about 25 percent fewer calories even without trying.

Most people have done it at least once in their lifetime. But did you know this habit of using a tiny utensil can help you lose weight?

Large servings with large utensils make it difficult for us to resist the urge to just binge through it all. In fact, we feel cheated when we're able to chow down through large servings in a few scoops. This makes us want to eat more. But small utensils cause us to slow down, and make us aware of how many scoops we've already taken in.

Cutting food up into smaller pieces may lead to more satiety than eating a larger piece of food with the same calories. A greater number of smaller pieces tricks the brain and gives it the appearance of a larger quantity.

Eat the following bite snacks one at a time to make you full faster:

- Nuts
- Cherry tomatoes
- Grapes
- Edamame
- Seeds
- Baby Brussel sprouts
- Berries
- Button mushrooms

How do you master the art of taking tiny bites?

- **Build the habit**: Commit to using tiny utensils for the next three days of dinner at home. Use cocktail forks, espresso spoons, and even baby spoons to start with. Use them for every part of the meal: from appetizers to the healthy parts.
- **Time yourself**: Time yourself when you finish these three meals from start to finish. Chances are, it takes you double the time to finish a regular serving. This allows you to listen to your hunger and pay attention to your fullness. It also gives you the opportunity to enjoy your food in smaller portions. When you chow down food in large gulps, you miss out on details like the texture and taste of the food.

When you master the art of taking tiny bites, you'll be able to taste all the food that you love minus the extra pounds.

Remember your pouch only works for portion control if you fill it. Snacking all day does not get food to hit the sides of your pouch and send signals that you are full. Start paying attention to gauging and measuring your bites and you will be back in business.

Planning a bariatric friendly meal that is healthy and tastes good at the same time can be tough. The bariatric life requires discipline and commitment, but it does not mean you need to put up with bland, tasteless meals.

Figure Sixty-Eight *(see next page)*

Making small changes can really add to or subtract from your calorie consumption during your bariatric journey.

BUILD A BARIATRIC FRIENDLY MEAL
PROTEIN + FAT + CARB

Choose one from each list to create a meal..........

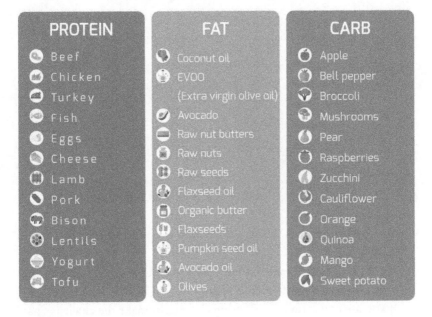

PROTEIN	FAT	CARB
Beef	Coconut oil	Apple
Chicken	EVOO	Bell pepper
Turkey	(Extra virgin olive oil)	Broccoli
Fish	Avocado	Mushrooms
Eggs	Raw nut butters	Pear
Cheese	Raw nuts	Raspberries
Lamb	Raw seeds	Zucchini
Pork	Flaxseed oil	Cauliflower
Bison	Organic butter	Orange
Lentils	Flaxseeds	Quinoa
Yogurt	Pumpkin seed oil	Mango
Tofu	Avocado oil	Sweet potato
	Olives	

Figure Sixty-Nine *(see next page)*

Though both these meals are considered healthy, depending on your bariatric goals, you need to make the modifications to increase protein, lower the carbs and calories, and be satiated after the meal. Rather than calorie counting, the table above demonstrates the impact ingredient manipulation can have on the overall calories in a meal.

***

Lose-Your-Regain Activity #twelve: Chopstick Challenge

Duration: twenty minutes

Slow down your meals and encourage small bites. This skill will make you aware when you are full and prevent the consumption of more calories than needed. Try using chopsticks to pace your meals.

- Buy a pair of chopsticks or utilize a leftover pair from a restaurant.

MEAL	MEAL 1	MEAL 2
	2 eggs ½ avocado	4 eggs 1 slice Ezekiel toast 1 whole avocado 1 apple 2 tbsp. peanut butter
Calories	260 calories	885 calories
Protein(g)	13 grams	41 grams
Carbs (g)	6 grams	59 grams
Fiber (g)	7 grams	23 grams
Fat(g)	25 grams	66 grams

- For three dinners in a row, utilize only chopsticks to eat your meal from start to finish.
- Notice how long it takes you to complete your meal, and if you paid more attention to the food on your plate.
- If you are comfortable with using chopsticks make the challenge harder by using your non-dominant hand to eat.

https://go.omadahealth.com

(Health, Omada. "The Omada Program". n.d)

***

Meet Melissa who got tired of being unhealthy and committed to making this a life-changing experience. She is working toward becoming an exercise specialist and helping other bariatric patients reach their weight loss goals. Read about her new-found energy as she jumps out and figures what else to conquer next. Expand your life as you shrink your body.

Figure Seventy *(see next page)*

Melissa: My name is Mellissa Johnson. I am thirty-six-years old and I am proud to say that I have lost 122 pounds. How did I do it? Well, here is my story. And hopefully through my journey, I can inspire and motivate you as well.

My weight loss journey began in 2015. I was at my heaviest weight, 280 pounds. And on a five-foot four-inch frame, that was not good. I was having shortness of breath after walking a few flights, my knees were always hurting, and my blood pressure and heart rate were elevated.

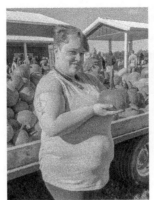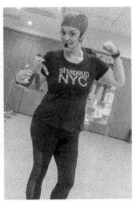

Coming from a family of heart disease, obesity, blood pressure, and diabetes, I was on the path to becoming another person in my family to having these issues.

Family gatherings always involved rice, beans, roasted pork, pasta, and some form of bread followed by desserts and coffee. And food was a way to get people together for a moment in one place at one time.

In junior high school, I began to see some weight issues, going up to about 150 by the eighth grade. In high school, I weighed in at 165 pounds. During my junior year, I enrolled in the Army Reserves Spilt Op program. I attended Basic training as a seventeen-year-old during the summer. To qualify for enrollment, I had to weigh in at 150 pounds. After a few weeks, I lost the needed weight and I was on my way. It was that summer, when I returned, that I was at my lowest, 145 pounds. If you don't know, military diets are strict, and the physical routines are rigorous. Nevertheless, I was happy and healthy.

In 2001, I met my first husband and the father of my now thirteen-year-old daughter. He was a cancer patient in remission for ten years at that time. And it was love at first sight. At that time, I weighed in at about 155 pounds., but my diet began to get off track. I was no longer eating what was healthy but what was convenient because we were always on the go.

In 2003, we planned on having a child together. However due to his extensive chemo and radiation at the age of sixteen, he was told he would not be able to have children. When he told me that, my heart broke and I was determined to give him a child. So, after extensive research, we found an In Vitro Fertilization (IVF) specialist and began the road of IVF treatments. The only issue was my weight. I was at 180 pounds and the specialist said if I wanted to have a better chance of conception, I had to lose weight. I had to get down to at least 165 pounds. My body went through a lot. From all the stress and injections and simply being pregnant at the very end of my pregnancy, I went up to a whopping 285 pounds. And after my daughter was born, I never broke the 200s.

Then in 2010, we received devastating news that would forever change my life. My husband's cancer came back and again my weight would take a turn. Over the following 10 months, until his passing, I hardly ate and slept. I wasn't getting the important nutrients. Finally, after a 11-month battle, long extensive hospital treatments and stay, he passed away and my world was crushed. Here I was, 27years-old with a 5-year-old and the man I vowed to be with for the rest of my life was gone. Why would I want to eat right? All I wanted and did do was eat because food and my daughter were the only things that brought me joy.

Over the next few years, I would continue to struggle with my weight. I topped the scale at 280 pounds. and I was on the verge of becoming diabetic. I had to do something. I tried different diets and I would lose weight but I would always gain back what I had lost and more. And because of all the weight, I felt uncomfortable and felt pain going to the gym. So, I just never went.

In 2015, I had enough. I wanted help. I needed help. The diets were not enough. I had heard of weight loss surgery but was reluctant to do it. Time and time again I would hear people say "Oh that's the easy way out for lazy people that don't want to work to get healthy. Just go on a diet." Well, I am here to tell you, that is far from the truth. It requires a lot of work to stay on track. Weight loss surgery does not take away addictions or cravings. It's not a fix all but a new lease on life. An option to take back your life.

I researched all the weight loss surgeries, from the lap band to bypass. I wanted to find a doctor that was knowledgeable in the field and had great success with his patients. That's when I was directed to my surgeon. With his guidance, compassion, and awesome staff, I chose to have the Vertical Sleeve Gastrectomy (commonly known as The Sleeve).

After all the hard work, doctors' visits, and paperwork, I got the call that would change my life forever. I got my surgery date, May 26, 2016 at six am. Things just got real. I was overcome by emotions. Finally, after years of battling obesity, I was going to get the help I needed to get my weight under control. From this point, I would be preparing to have surgery.

My journey from the date I had surgery to the present day has been nothing short of amazing. Yes, there were days I question if I made the right decision. There were days I would compare my journey to that of others and I felt I was a complete failure. I was worried that I would fail as a patient. That I would not lose weight at all, or even to the expectations of my surgeon. I was so wrong.

It took me two years, but I am proud to say that I lost a total of 122 pounds. That's right 122 pounds. A whole other person. My life has been so amazing since May 26, 2016. I can play with my nieces, run on a treadmill for fifteen minutes straight with no breaks, and I'm in the gym four times a week. What's even better, I have inspired my family to get healthier and even some of my clients.

Portion control is something that takes time to get down and get used to. There are so many ways to portion control. In the beginning, I went to Dollar Tree and bought the small little Betty Crocker containers. I would pre-measure the food that would go in the containers. Trust me, it may not seem like a lot, but when you've had 80% of your stomach removed, four ounces can feel like a thanksgiving meal. I did that for about six months. My fiancé then purchased a digital food scale for me that showed all the nutritional values I needed to stay on target with my macros. I would then weigh out as well as measure my food and place it in a container.

Exercise is a percentage of the success in weight loss. As I got further into my journey, I decided I had to get into the gym. So, my fiancé and I went to a local gym and joined as a couple. Part of my success with my exercise has a lot to do with pre-planning workouts. I also created an accountability team where I would check in with a group of my fellow weight loss and non-weight loss buddies.

I can honestly say that this journey has been nothing but amazing and has taught me a lot and has literally given me my life back. I have done and accomplished so much: from losing 122 pounds to now being on my way to becoming a certified personal trainer, fitness nutritional specialist, and group fitness instructor. But I really want to give a world of thanks to the man that stood by my side, loving me at every size and through all the ups and downs, fears, and joys. Pushing me to keep going when I just wanted to give up. To my loving fiancé and best friend Antonio, thank you for never doubting me and being that cheerleader and constant support.

In closing, I want to say that if you are fearful of having the surgery or have people saying that you'll never succeed, block them out. Block out the negativity and take back what's rightfully yours – your health and life. Surround yourself with as much positive and strong support as possible by joining support groups and meet-ups of fellow weight loss patients. Take your time and have patience with the process. Remember masterpieces take time to create. And always remember, you are worth it.

Chapter Thirteen:
Interactive Weight Loss Tools

*"Life expectancy would grow by leaps and bounds
if green vegetables smelled as good as bacon."*
–Doug Larson

Bliss Out with Tech

Technology can either be a good thing or a bad thing. It has been frequently blamed for sedentary lives, but should not have to be a reason to sit still. Using it as a motivator to spark behavior change and reach health and fitness goals, bariatric patients stay engaged longer.

"Interactive health" is all about you, the consumer, and your everyday engagement in your wellbeing, your health, and your weight loss journey. There are various gaming, social networking tools, and consumer applications that can engage and keep you on track (Tofighi et al,2018,715-731).

Health insurance companies may soon start selling policies that track health and fitness data through smart phones or wearable devices. Policy holders may get premier discounts and other perks on hitting exercise targets tracked by their Fitbit or apple watch. It is a win-win situation in the long run, where you are incentivized to adopt healthier habits and insurance companies collect more premiums while paying less in claims.

The following devices if used correctly could help you lose weight:

- Smart Scales
- Fitness trackers
- Weight loss trackers
- Electronic water bottles
- Game consoles

Smart Scales

Monitoring your weight is no fun, but then to lose it you need to watch it. Regular scales can be replaced with smart bathroom scales which, besides measuring weight, also give you a rundown of your body mass index (BMI), fat percentage, and muscle mass.

The difference between a smart scale and a regular one is that it recognizes its owner and can tell other family members apart. It is easy to synch with your smart phone and follows your weight changes very closely.

In addition to measuring weight, smart scales calculate fat percentage and BMI. Additional benefits are having support and motivation, where the gadget keeps track of your accomplishments and advises on improvement.

Fitness Trackers

Fitness trackers monitor your daily steps and offer an effective way to stay on your toes all the time. Setting your goals for the day helps you to stay active and hit those goals. Daily updates engage the users to compete with themselves, and keep their morale high.

This is the most popular and best known of health gadgets where a motion sensor keeps track of your steps 24/7. It is an interactive coach who pushes you to walk more to reach your dream weight. Based on information that can be input into the database, these devices also calculate the calories burned and the possible consequences on your weight loss journey.

Some trackers identify different types of activity levels and have a built-in heart monitor. Additional apps can help you watch your diet and count your caloric intake. They can connect you to your nutritionist or fitness trainer for results. Other trackers can calculate the calories in local supermarkets by scanning the barcodes when you are food shopping. Certain devices monitor your sleeping patterns along with your heart rate and electrocardiogram (EKG) changes. Adequate sleep is imperative to prevent weight regain and monitoring it can help you make changes for a good night's sleep. Swimming fitness trackers, a waterproof version, helps you keep track underwater. Smart watches try to interact between a fitness tracker and the running shoes of famous manufacturers. It motivates the wearer to run regularly and gives advice on the proper techniques of running. It considers the landscape changes and compares results of previous runs.

Weight Loss Trackers

These gadgets analyze muscle to fat tissue ratio in the body. They measure the muscle and fat tissue and gives detailed statistics on it. In addition to motivating constant physical activity, they help to keep you on your toes.

Electronic Water Bottles

Hydration is vital, in addition to eating well, right to losing regained weight. Electronic water bottles are compatible with Android and iOS platforms. These intelligent bottles use an app to calculate your daily personal fluid intake, guiding your frequency and volume of consumption throughout the day. In addition to pointing out flaws, the bottle will help you adjust your hydration routine to stimulate the loss of weight.

Game Consoles

Fitness video games promotes activity without leaving your living room. The options make it an ideal solution when one is fatigued. These workout games help people stick to a routine where consistency also plays a vital role.

Virtual workout systems help you lose weight while playing simulation games. Virtual coaches demonstrate exercises that you repeat. Each squat or lunge you do is worth a certain number of points, which are calculated at the end of each session. Although the coach is virtual, the workout is very demanding and is very popular with individuals trying to lose weight.

Using Social Media to Lose Weight

Millions of people all around the world spend a lot of time on social media. For many, it is the first thing they open in the morning and the last thing they look at before going to bed. It is a great platform to update yourself on what's happening with your network.

While some people criticize the negative effects of excess social media use, you can also choose to use the platform to create positive impacts in your life. Social media is not only a venue to communicate and update your life status. This can also be an avenue for you to lose weight (Chou et al,2014,314-323).

When you log on, there are many people interacting and having conversations with each other on fitness, weight loss, and health. You can take advantage of this to help you lose weight and connect with others on similar journeys. This can be a relatively good tool for you to stay motivated, reach success, and remain accountable for your actions. All these things ultimately facilitate behavior change (Koball et al,2018,1897-1902).

Here are some concrete ways that social media can help your weight loss goals:

Inspiration

Social media sites feature inspirational photos that can serve as a motivation for you. These photo rich social media platforms allow you to discover boards and images of people with their fitness goals. These visual reminders can help you push harder and get yourself to the gym.

Fitness Guide

Social media can also be a great source of exercise routines, tips, and advice. There are many credible fitness professionals who share their stories, feature videos of their diet and exercise routine, as well as provide different recommendations to guide people struggling to be healthier.

Communities

Another great thing about social media is the presence of communities grounded on common interests. There are already a lot of groups that are geared towards supporting each other in their fitness journey.

They usually share gym routines, diets that work best for them, and encourage others. This can be your support group that will help you push harder. Participants find themselves in the process of building communities in the process, and reaching outcomes that would never be possible on their own.

Sharing your fitness journey with your family, friends, and network can help support you and urge you forward. Interacting with others who share the same goals as you leads to accountability and successful weight loss. Surrounding yourself with weight loss surgery patients, virtually helps you carry out your healthy behaviors.

If you are still not on social media, here are some popular social media platforms that you can consider:

Facebook is usually a friends and family platform where people share their journey and get much needed support. Triumphs and frustrations are shared on your news feed. Facebook enables you to put your best foot forward, boost self-esteem, and celebrate your success with family and friends. Don't forget to adjust privacy settings if needed.

Twitter provides motivating feedback from fellow users and is the perfect platform to announce your weight loss goals, run a 10K and watch the "likes" pop up. It is also ideal for finding articles on weight loss topics and the latest news. Popular hashtags like #health, #weight loss, #fitness, and #exercise come in very handy. Twitter is an effective tool for weight loss, due to increased access to information, social support, and progress in real time.

Pinterest is a favorite platform for inspirational quotes, recipes, and photo-focused visual inspiration. Create digital vision boards on Pinterest for each one of your healthy interests like slow cooker recipes, jogging inspirations, and at-home exercises.

Instagram utilizes photos of before and after weight loss journeys. Be aware that, though scrolling through drool-worthy photos of food may seem harmless, it may trigger indulgence of food and exacerbate physical hunger.

Apps and text message services send notifications reminding you to eat right and exercise. These messages serve as a virtual coach who checks in with you and keeps you focused. If you are having trouble sticking to the protocols, invest in an app or device that provides gentle reminders and daily feedback.

Figure Seventy-One

Social Media Saboteurs

 · Avoid negativity that may come from making your personal life more public.

 · Keep progress positive.

 · Do not compare yourself to others.

 · Don't listen to the trolls.

 · You oversee your privacy and decide what is best for you.

 · Spending too much time on social media.

 · Blindly following fitness influencers.

 · Watch out for unhelpful or dangerous advice.

Helpful Apps
- The Stop, Breathe and Think app offers guided meditations to suit your current state of mind. Free app: www.stopbreathethink.com
- You select a weight loss challenge based on how much you want to bet. Losing at least 4% of your body weight leads to you winning the money you bet on yourself. www.dietbet.com
- Personalized or group tabata - based interval workouts with in - app coaching.
- www.activexapp.com
- This app tracks your sleep cycle via sound and movement analysis, minimizing exhaustion and grogginess when waking up. www.sleepcycle.com
- App uses science-based strategies to increase overall well-being and life satisfaction. https://happify.com
- This app is for runners where you select how many miles you want to run and the app generates a route for you. www.mapmyrun.com
- Track your food intake either by scanning barcodes, or manually entering calories. https://loseit.com
- This app brings the benefits of a spin class to your phone. Choose your instructor, class length and playlist. www.cyclecast.com

Apps from the app store
- **Studio**: If you are running for weight loss.
- **Sleep cycle**: For sleep issues.
- **Interval timer**: High intensity interval training.
- **Aaptiv**: If you have trouble sticking to one workout.
- **Mindful Eating Tracker**: Improve your relationship with food.
- **Lose it**: Track your daily calories.
- **Myfitnesspal**: Portion sizes confusion.
- **Healthyout**: Need to find a healthy restaurant.
- **Muse**: For meditation

***

Lose-Your-Regain Activity # thirteen: Skill: Make An Emotional Eating Emergency Kit

When feelings fuel cravings, an emotional eating emergency kit (E.E.E.K). will help. You have two parts of your brains that are constantly in conflict, the emotional side and the logical side. While the logical side will always know that you want to stay on track and keep that weight off long-term after bariatric surgery, it's the emotional side that just really loves brownies. You may find yourself using snacks to comfort yourself emotionally. This creates a vicious cycle of eating, feeling guilty about it, and then eating more.

One way to fight emotional eating is to fight your feelings with feelings. An Emotional Eating Emergency Kit (also known as EEEK!) is a collection of items that represent your heartfelt reasons for wanting to stay at your goal weight. When negative feelings fuel cravings for unfriendly snacks, consulting your EEEK! can help defuse them with positive motivation.

How to Complete This Skill:
- Get an empty container like a shoe box or anything about that size
- Start filling it with things that remind you of why you want to stay at your goal weight and why staying on track is important to you. Here are some ideas to get you started:
  - Photos of your kids, or anyone with whom you want to live a long and healthy life with.
  - Photos of a role model whose strength and dedication inspires you.
  - Write a note to yourself about why you deserve to stay healthy even after the honey moon period, why you will never go back to your pre-surgical weight, how you will run that 5K and/or how your life will be different and worthwhile when you get to your goal.
  - Write out a motivational mantra or inspiring poem.
  - Place a stress relief ball in there.
  - Write out a list of other feel-good, distracting activities that can give you instant relief, like calling a specific friend, spending time with your pet, or watching a few minutes of your favorite comedian on YouTube.
- Place the box in your kitchen cabinet or work desk right next to where you keep your snacks, so when you get hungry and are at risk of emotional eating, you'll be able to reflect before you dig in.

https://go.omadahealth.com
Health,Omada. "The Omada Program."

***

Meet Maria who knew that sleeve gastrectomy was the tool she needed to turn her weight loss failures into a weight loss success story. She realized that if she did not go through the surgery, she would always be unhealthy, angry and miserable which she did not want. Read about how she deliberately chose a healthier pattern to her life and gained control over her eating. Be deliberate in your choices today.

Figure Seventy-Two *(see next page)*

Maria: To tell you where I am, I must tell you where I come from and how I got to my Bari-Birthday, June of 2016. I am a middle child born into a Spanish family. My mother, a nutritionist by education, always made sure we were fed. Even though she worked, she came home to make dinner and have lunch ready for the next school day.

My mother's cooking was not any different than most Hispanics – a small size portion of chicken or beef and a larger serving of rice and/or beans, some sort of fried plantain, yucca or

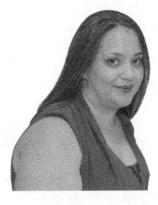
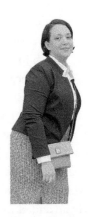

potatoes. Some nights there was an appearance of a small serving of vegetable or salad. Birthday parties or any type of celebration meant food galore. In Spanish families, you can never have too much. Food was huge and we always had an excuse to get together and celebrate.

Growing up, I took up basketball and dance and managed to always be an appropriate size up until the end of high school. As my activity level changed and my eating habits stayed consistent my weight began to slowly increase.

I found myself thinking about how it was possible for my mom, the nutritionist, to allow me and most of my family to be overweight. She herself has struggled constantly with her weight and weight loss. She was always on the last fad diet and would try to get us to go along with her but that was no easy task. The diet I remember most vividly was the cabbage diet, because of the disgusting smell. According to her it involved eating cabbage soup at each meal and that would guarantee weight loss. As you might imagine, our little apartment in Elmhurst stunk because of the smell of the cabbage, yet my mother was determined. She would lose a pound here and there and gain five the following weekend.

Looking back, I can honestly say that in all the yo-yo dieting my mother did, she never included exercise into the regime. After our family meal, we would sit around the television and wait for bed time to come.

I know that my weight gain is not my mother's fault because I chose to put the fork in my mouth and I stepped away from the physical activities I had been doing prior to the weight gain. This is something that I realized when I was past the point of no return at over 200 pounds and a junior in college. Nonetheless I did not make a change until much after. Instead I owned my large life. I had all types of come backs for anyone that commented on it. I was not fat. I was fluffy. I was not fat. I was going to die happy and on a full stomach.

After my marriage and multiple pregnancies, I was as big as I ever got and as big as I will ever be. I was 268 pounds at 5 feet 5 inches. During this time, I was also a stay at home mom that practically lived in the kitchen. Making countless meals because food was love, so I thought. And I lived to eat. I went to sleep planning the next day's meals, which included homemade desserts on some nights.

My complicated pregnancy in 2010 was a result of a newly acquired and chronic high blood pressure diagnosis and sleep apnea. The high blood pressure resulted in my son not being able to develop at the normal pace and caused an early delivery. I had to deliver at seven months after being hospitalized for three weeks. He was born in the seventh percentile which means he was under three pounds. He passed after five days of an infection he acquired in the NICU. If it wasn't for my medical issues he would not have been in the NICU. The sadness and emptiness was drowned in food and added to the continued weight gain.

Fast forward to 2015, after countless doctors telling me to lose weight, I asked my obstetrician-gynecologist (OBGYN) about weight loss surgery. It was the first time I had contemplated that I need to change my life, my eating habits, and my body. She referred me to my surgeon and I made the appointment. At this point, I had a lot of questions regarding the surgery. I had many doubts if it was for me. I remember going to the consultation and having all my questions answered but leaving still with doubts. The moment it all changed was the moment my husband snapped a picture of me and the kids and I saw the mom in the picture and I was disgusted. I will never forget the lump I felt in my stomach. As I took it in, I vowed that that would be my last fat girl pic.

I scheduled another appointment with my surgeon and this time I went in there knowing that this was going to be the decision that changed my life. I took all the information that was given to me and headed out on my mission. My mission to regain my life, to have a longer and healthier life, and to be the best mom ever. There were so many skeptics on this road, my mother being the first and biggest one. Talk about raining on my parade. She researched and managed to find so many negative views about this surgery and constantly challenged my decision. It was not the easiest of roads, but thanks to some individuals that I met along the way I was able to re-educate myself and re-program my brain for success and educate even my mom. Yes, there are many negatives out there but those negatives only come into play if you do not do as you are told.

Soon enough it was my Bari-Birthday, June 7, 2016. The morning of my surgery I went to the hospital all prepared to have my surgery that I worked hard for. I was dressed in my surgical gown and got a last-minute phone call that the insurance had not approved my surgery and I would have to wait. I was devastated, but then the office stepped in and worked their magic, and once again I was back on track and ready to head into surgery.

According to my surgeon, my surgery was a success. The day before surgery all my medicine was discontinued and I have never had to go back to it. No more high blood pressure. Now it was my turn to make it last that way. I followed each instruction carefully and precisely. There was protein everywhere once I came home. I had little medicine like cups in every room. As soon as the timer went off, I took a sip. The beginning was easy. Then it gets boring. Just like the liquid diet we are required to follow pre-surgery, it's the same for post-surgery. How much more liquid could I take? We were about to find out. I had protein soups, sugar-free jello, protein drinks, protein water, protein popsicles, protein everything. If it didn't have a high level of protein it wasn't going into my mouth. I had to stick to this. I had to do it right. I kept flipping back to that picture my husband took. I wanted nothing to do with that person.

After each check in with my surgeon I received good news. Each time I had lost more and more weight. Soon enough the holidays were approaching. The thought of all that food was nerve racking but the "picture" was my saving grace. I was down ninety-nine pounds in six months!!! The secret to losing the ninety nine pounds is not so much a secret. It's food preparation and sticking to the protein, protein, protein rule.

I prepared as many meals as possible. My whole family adjusted to my form of eating, the protein portion always being larger on all the plates served in my home. My plate was solely protein but the children and hubby got their vegetable sides. My house went practically carb-less for a real long time. I made my meals to take with me to work and places where I believed might not have the best options for me. I packed my protein drinks for days out with the kids, and packed snacks that I could have, like sugar - free jello and pudding. Pasta and rice were a thing of the past or a thing at someone else's house. As I lost my weight, my husband did as well. My children learned about healthier eating with my diet.

I slowly became more active. I was sleeping better and had happier days. I was making it past the couch potato time. Traded the couch in for the park with the kids, the college track, and bicycle riding. During the colder months, I get out with our family dog more and try to pop in a Zumba video. This year I did my first color run.

Maintaining the weight loss is my purpose in life now. This still means food preparation and when I am unable to making the right decisions, I look for beef stew and baked chicken at the local buffet by work for lunch. Dinner is made at home each night. Once a month I will make a pasta for the family, but I will remove my portion of protein before I incorporate the pasta with the meat. I will make burgers but make sure mine is bun-less. Eating out means looking at the appetizers and seeing what has the lowest amount of carbs and most amount of protein. Treats include low sodium beef jerky and pork rinds. I always have almonds and cashews around as a snack. Breakfast is always an egg with bacon or sausage.

Post-surgery also brought some marital issues. My husband did not like the new attention I was receiving and there were numerous conversations over it. I was only appreciating the compliments that even my mother was giving me. It took a lot for both him and me to adjust to this attention.

On most days, I still feel like the fat girl and I must remind myself how far I have come. My bat wings, clapping thighs, and over-hung belly are a constant reminder of where I never want to go back. These are now my stripes to wear with honor. I have officially gone back to a two-piece bathing suit for the beach, and to wearing shorts, skirts, and dresses in the summer since my thighs now clap instead of rubbing. Short hair doesn't matter since I don't have to hide my fat face.

Bariatric surgery saved my life and I must keep saving it every day with the choices I make. Only the person who went through this process knows what it means to them. And only they can continue making the correct decisions to insure it. I have chosen to use my surgery as a tool for myself and as an example for anyone around who is contemplating it.

Chapter Fourteen:
Never Look Back

"In order to change we must be sick and tired of being sick and tired."
– Unknown

Use Failure to Your Advantage

As per Dr. Travis Bradberry the author of the best-selling book *"Emotional Intelligence 2.0",* one of the biggest roadblocks to weight loss success is the fear of failure. When one fears of failing and going back to the pre-surgical weight, that is worse than failure itself (Bradberry, T & Greaves, J. 2009).

A successful response to weight regain is the way you approach it. In a recent study published in the *Journal of Experimental Social Psychology,* researchers discovered that success in the face of failure arises from focusing on results rather than trying not to fail. When you put all your energy on trying to avoid failure, you fail far more often than someone who optimistically focuses on their goals (Fotuhi O et al, 2014).

Despite it sounding easy, it's very hard to do when the consequences of weight loss failure are severe (restarting medications, going back on the CPAP machine). Positive feedback from family and friends during this period increases one's chances of losing the regained weight because it fuels the same optimism one experiences when focusing solely on their goals.

So, what puts people who let their failures derail them in a separate category than from those who use failure to their advantage? It is what you do to get to your goals, and the rest is what you think during your journey there.

Every single action you take during the period of losing the regained weight is critical to your ability to get back on track. The implications are huge for how people around you view you and your actions. Eight actions you adopt when you find yourself back where you started that will enable you to succeed and surround yourself with positivity.

- **Be aware of yourself.** If you see yourself regaining weight, don't cross your fingers and hope that it will go away by ignoring it. When others point out your regain, that one step backwards turns into two. Staying quiet and not doing anything about it makes people wonder why you are not standing up for yourself, and they're likely to attribute this to either you giving up or you being ignorant of it.
- **Know the difference between an explanation and an excuse**. Owning your mistakes can actually put you on the right path. It shows you have confidence in your abilities, you are accountable, and have integrity. Make sure to stick to the facts. "I regained weight because I started eating carbs" is a reason. "I regained weight because I have no time to exercise" is an excuse.
- **Plan to fix things.** You accept you made a mistake, but what are you planning on doing about it? The next step is critical. Instead of giving up, or waiting for someone else to clean up your mess, plan to offer your own solutions. It's even better if you can tell your nutritionist or surgeon or psychologist the specific steps that you've already taken to get things back on track.
- **Plan for prevention.** While you figure out a plan for fixing things, also have a plan for how you'll avoid making the same mistake in the future. That's the best way to reassure YOURSELF that positive things will come out of your failure.
- **Get back on track.** It is vital that failure does not make you timid. Having this mindset will suck you in and weaken you every time you slip up. Once you have taken the time to absorb the lessons of your failure, get right back on track and try again. Prolonging this action will create bad feelings and increases the chances of permanent spiraling. Your attitude is just as important as the actions you take when facing weight loss failure. Use failure to your advantage and stay optimistic, be persistent and have a positive perspective.
- **Perspective** is the most important factor when handling weight regain after bariatric surgery. Patients who plateau after weight loss are more likely to blame the regain on something that they are responsible for – the wrong course of action they took or a specific oversight that they kept repeating—rather than who they are. People who are bad at handling a speedbump like weight regain tend to blame their current state on their laziness, lack of motivation, or some other personal quality, implying that they had no control over the situation. They belong to the category of people who avoid any future risk-taking.
- **Optimism** is another factor of people who bounce back from weight regain. This sense of optimism is what keeps them from feeling like weight regain

is a permanent condition. Instead, they tend to see each pound lost as a building block to their ultimate weight loss success because of the knowledge it provides.

- **Persistence.** It's optimism along with action. When people around you say, "I'm done" and decide to quit, a persistent person shakes off those feelings and keeps going. Persistent people are successful at rising from failure since their optimism never dies.

***

Bringing It All Together

Looking at yourself as a failure is a product of your perspective. What one person considers a "never to be won" battle, another sees as a minor setback. The most positive aspect is that you can change how failure is perceived in order to use it to better yourself.

Barriers to Weight Loss

Certain potential barriers to consider when getting back on the weight loss track are:

1: What are your sources of joy?

Are you always thinking about food and looking forward to mealtimes since that gives you immense pleasure and joy? If so, how do you plan on replacing it? Gardening? Taking a walk?

2: How social are you?

Sticking to portion sizes, having the willpower, and overeating is harder if you are dating or socializing. Learn to make excuses when eating out or be less social for a while. It will be totally worth it.

3: Is your family on board?

Finding yourself in a family environment where everyone has an opinion is tough on losing weight. Families make demands on your time, fill your refrigerator with foods you need to stay away from, dislike change, and may have different goals than yours. Be patient and nice when getting everyone around you on board.

4: Do you have the time?

Getting back on track and losing regained weight is likely to take more of your time than not doing it. Nobody has infinite time or energy. It is easier to order take- out than cook a meal, easier to sit on the couch than exercise, to sit up late working than get a good night's sleep.

5: Are you addressing the underlying problems?

After bariatric surgery, people find that they literally become a different person, even if the weight comes off slowly. They believe people treat them differently. This process of losing weight may not fix all the problems you would like it to, but the set of changes you experience as a result will be hugely valuable across many areas of life. It is a strange phenomenon that weight loss surgery rapidly increases a person's chances of separating or getting divorced. Though the reasons are hard to understand, it seems the partners have difficulty in adjusting to the new person.

***

The True Meaning of Self-Care

Self-care is a good thing, and we all need it. But it can be a challenge to know how to take care of ourselves, even when we know that self-care is outside of our programming. We are good at taking care of others, but the knowledge on how to take care of ourselves eludes us.

What is self-care anyway? Apart from taking care of your most basic needs, like food, clothing, and shelter, taking good care of one's self is situational and personal. It requires personal responsibility to not let other people control us. It also requires personal responsibility to not take a backseat to other people. Our sense of self comes first and foremost always, and the others are secondary.

How can we take better care of ourselves?

If you want to take better care of yourself, you must know yourself. What are your strengths? What are your weaknesses? What are you reliant upon? What are your needs? What are your wants? This is a personal journey of trial and error.

But that's not an overnight journey. We have blind spots and we have flaws that we don't want to accept, and these often hinder us from understanding the true meaning of self-care. Therefore, most people work with coaches and therapists because it helps to identify these blind spots and flaws, when they're pointed out by other people. And yes, it can be difficult to admit to your own blind spots and flaws.

Self-care is a dynamic process. We learn how to manage ourselves overtime and get better at it with constant practice. Self-care is doing what truly serves you now. The simple act of relieving stress is already a practice of self-care. Going out for a walk instead of eating junk food is a practice of self-care. Self-care is growing yourself to become a better version of yourself, one step at a time.

***

What's with the Attitude?

It is very normal to beat yourself up. Mistakes do happen and nobody is perfect. You might call yourself a perfectionist but you might still be far from perfect during your bariatric journey. The only thing you can do is pick yourself up, give yourself a pep talk and move on. Every day you wake up is a second chance. Look for solutions to your problems or they will end up becoming excuses.

Figure Seventy-Three

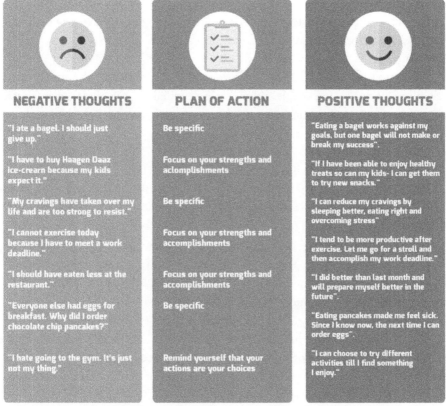

NEGATIVE THOUGHTS	PLAN OF ACTION	POSITIVE THOUGHTS
"I ate a bagel. I should just give up."	Be specific	"Eating a bagel works against my goals, but one bagel will not make or break my success".
"I have to buy Haagen Daaz ice-cream because my kids expect it."	Focus on your strengths and aclomplishments	"If I have been able to enjoy healthy treats so can my kids- I can get them to try new snacks."
"My cravings have taken over my life and are too strong to resist."	Be specific	"I can reduce my cravings by sleeping better, eating right and overcoming stress"
"I cannot exercise today because I have to meet a work deadline."	Focus on your strengths and accomplishments	"I tend to be more productive after exercise. Let me go for a stroll and then accomplish my work deadline."
"I should have eaten less at the restaurant."	Focus on your strengths and accomplishments	"I did better than last month and will prepare myself better in the future".
"Everyone else had eggs for breakfast. Why did I order chocolate chip pancakes?"	Be specific	"Eating pancakes made me feel sick. Since I know now, the next time I can order eggs".
"I hate going to the gym. It's just not my thing."	Remind yourself that your actions are your choices	"I can choose to try different activities till I find something I enjoy."

https://go.omadahealth.com Health, Omada. "The Omada Program."

***

Rules and Tools to Maintain Your Weight Loss

Once you are at your goal weight, you have graduated to the maintenance phase that will continue for life.

Do you love your pet? You feed them and groom them well. You give them a lot of attention and indulge them on a regular basis. Treat yourself the same way. Value, respect and nourish yourself. Cherish your accomplishments and never put yourself on the back burner. Commit to never abusing your body and increase the self-care to reflect in real life. Some rules and tools to follow during your maintenance phase are:

Eat breakfast

Eating within thirty minutes of waking up is a good habit to develop for life. Skipping breakfast activates the adrenal glands to produce an emergency hormone that tells your body to go into starvation mode and stockpile the fat. Lose the fat and keep the muscle. Start eating your breakfast.

Snack Stash

If you get hungry or it's a few hours since your last meal, rather than reaching out for the wrong foods, have a stash of healthy snacks in your bag, your car, your desk, and your freezer. Be ready for emergencies.

Keep sipping

Hydration is an essential habit and enhances your metabolism and helps with weight loss. It flushes out toxins and prevents dehydration. Sip all day to reach your limit of at least sixty four ounces instead of trying to catch up right before you go to bed.

Real food, real weight loss

The ingredient list is what matters. Watch out for fake sugars and fake fats. If you are not familiar with the ingredients stay away from them. No matter what you eat within the bariatric protocols, make sure it is real food.

Five meals a day

Three meals with two snacks on every day of your weight loss journey will keep your metabolism working. Rotate the content of your snacks every few days. To keep your body metabolism guessing, rotate two days of protein snacks, with two days of healthy fat snacks and two days of fruit-based snacks.

Slow cook when busy

When you are pressed for time, prep the slow cooker the night before. Plug it in and turn it on before work. Look up slow cooker recipes and treat yourself and your family to delicious hot dinners. The temptation of frozen dinners, takeout, or skipping a meal will fly out of the window.

Prep time

Prep your meals for the week ahead on the weekend. Mentally chart out your breakfast, dinners, and snacks. Use leftovers as lunch. Making a soup and marinating chicken or fish can cut your cooking time in half during the week. Make it a part of your routine and you will have time to exercise also.

Exercise

Exercise every day for a minimum of thirty minutes. Rotate cardio, strength training, and healing (yoga and Pilates) exercises. Increase the mitochondria in your cells and burn more fat.

Stay away

Avoid sugar, alcohol, bagels, bread, corn, potatoes, and processed foods. Do you really want to go back to killing your progress? Slipping occasionally changes to two to three times a week, and before you know it a bad habit has evolved.

Use the freezer

Chop up your vegetables and fruit and freeze them for days when you are running out of time. It is easy and less stressful to make a quick meal when food is pre-made. Check your freezer inventory on a regular basis to rotate foods and reduce wastage.

Stress away

Do not let stress get the better of you. Take care of yourself, learn to say "NO," breathe deeply, and relax. This is crucial to keeping the weight at bay.

***

Rethink the Rules of Weight Loss after Bariatric Surgery

Old Rule: **Exercise to burn calories**.

New Rule: Exercise to build your fitness level and maximize your metabolism. Increasing the number of your mitochondria by exercise, helps you raise your metabolism, burn more calories, and lose more weight.

Old Rule: **Losing weight is about changing your body**.

New Rule: Losing weight after bariatric surgery is about changing your life. To lose weight and keep it off long- term, both your body and mind must be on board.

Old Rule: **Fat makes you fat.**

New Rule: Good fats are good for you. Understand the difference between bad fats (found in processed foods) and good fats like nuts, seeds, and fish. Eating a moderate amount of good fat keeps your blood sugars under control and keeps you full longer, both of which have a direct impact on successful weight loss and maintenance.

Old Rule: **Count your calories.**

New Rule: Upgrade your calories. More than the quantity of calories you eat, driving weight loss, it's the nature and quality of these calories that matter for the body to function optimally. Feed your body foods that have a low glycemic load (GL) and high phytonutrient index (PI), like beans, nuts, olive oil, and vegetables. While a low GL meal slows down the conversion of carbs to sugar, it also stops the trigger of metabolic signals that promote hunger and weight gain. High PI foods heal and regulate the metabolism.

Old Rule: **To lose weight, diet.**

New Rule: To lose weight, nourish your body.

When you diet, or skip meals to lose weight, there might be a temporary weight loss, but ultimately it puts the body in a "fat conservation" mode. The deprivation diet sets up a "just-until-I-lose-this-weight" mentality, which is an enemy of long-lasting weight loss.

***

Bariatric post ops tend to lose their teeth years after bariatric surgery due to bone loss from the jaw area. The body goes through tremendous change after bariatric surgery and broken teeth are a side effect of mineral deficiencies.

Dental Health after Bariatric Surgery

Life after bariatric surgery places a lot of restrictions on the bariatric patient. In addition to spreading their meals throughout the day, they need to chew food well before they swallow it.

Gastric restriction can induce chronic vomiting, gastro esophageal reflux, and stomach ulcers. Clinical studies published in the *International Dental Journal* have shown that after bariatric surgery:

- 79% of patients reported vomiting as their most frequent problem.
- 73% stuck to their pre-operative dental hygiene habits.
- 37% reported cravings for sweet foods.
- 37% reported major sensitivity of teeth

Stillwell, David. "Obesity Complicates Dental Health." *Obesity Action Coalition*. https://www.obesityaction.org/community/article.../obesity-complicates-dental-health/

Overeating after bariatric surgery causes distention of the gastric pouch which in turn leads to reflux and regurgitation. When teeth are exposed to gastric juices at a pH. of 1.2, tooth structure starts dissolving. (7.0 is the neutral pH). This leads to dental erosion where patients constantly complain of sensitivity to cold and hot foods. Craving for sweets compounds the situation, leading to a frenzy of oral bacteria producing more acid.

As per David Stillwell, DDS an associate professor at University of Arkansas, dental erosion after bariatric surgery can be prevented by:

- Making wise food choices.
- Eating small meals.
- Controlling heartburn and reflux with prescription medications.
- Taking calcium and vitamin D supplementation on a consistent basis.

Prescription drugs come with a price tag and cause xerostomia (dry mouth), which might have major dental consequences like:

- Taste alterations or dysgeusia.
- Mucositis or chronic irritation and inflammation of oral tissue.
- Dental decay.
- Erosion.
- Interference with normal swallowing patterns

Stillwell, David. "Obesity Complicates Dental Health." *Obesity Action Coalition*. https://www.obesityaction.org/community/article.../obesity-complicates-dental-health/

Dr. Stillwell outlines a **five-point strategy plan** to control your dental destiny:

- Modify your daily diet by eating more seeds, nuts, spinach and seafood, which starves decay - producing bacteria and reduces acid levels in the mouth. Reduce acidic foods like bread, pasta, coffee, chocolate, and fruit juices.

- Moisturize and lubricate the mouth with increased consumption of fluoridated drinking water. Include six to ten grams every day of Xylitol sweetened products to reduce dental plaque. This increases natural saliva flow. Use caution with the usage of polyol sweeteners like sorbitol, mannitol, and xylitol. If these sugar substitutes are taken in large amounts it can lead to osmotic diarrhea in bariatric patients.
- Neutralize the environment by increasing the pH of the mouth. Brush your teeth with a coating of baking soda on your toothpaste for a quick neutralizing treatment.
- Re-mineralize damaged tooth surfaces by using fluoride pastes, gels, and rinses. This tends to enhance the re-mineralization of the tooth surface and inhibit bacterial metabolism.
- Disinfect your mouth to reduce disease causing oral bacteria. Effectively rinsing with Listerine mouthwash for one minute disrupts dental plaque and is the best method for bacterial control.

Stillwell, David. "Obesity Complicates Dental Health." *Obesity Action Coalition*. https://www.obesityaction.org/community/article.../obesity-complicates-dental-health/

***

Lose-Your-Regain Activity # fourteen: Commit Yourself to a Fresh Start

Refocus your efforts to stay healthy and step on the scale for seven days straight.
- **Time**: Weigh yourself at the same time every day.
- **Place:** Keep your scale in the same place to get consistent results.
- **Method**: Weigh in naked or in your underwear.
- **Trigger**: Remind yourself to track your weight by choosing an activity you do daily like after my shower or before I brush my teeth.
- **Start**: Pick your time, place, method, and trigger, and get going.

The goal is to see a downward trend. Don't fixate too much on the numbers. The reason you weigh yourself every day is to remind yourself that you will never go back to where you came from and to recommit every day to eating better and exercising consistently.

https:/go.omadahealth.com

Health, Omada. "The Omada Program."

***

Meet Dana who is excited to be living again! She still puts in the work every day and is determined to keep her life on track with a healthy lifestyle. Read about how she overcomes her fears and worries and is aware of the reality that she can maintain her weight loss. Remember fears and worries are not facts. Fight back.

Figure Seventy-Four

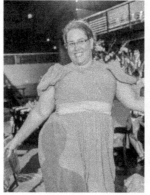
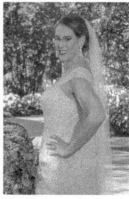

Dana: I was always the "big girl!" Born a normal size and weight, I was six feet tall at the age of twelve. My doctor used to tell me I was overweight and needed to watch what I ate. I had trouble finding clothing that fit me at age twelve. I was comfortable with my weight, confident, loud, and funny. I had a difficult relationship with my mom, growing up where weight was always an issue.

I used food for comfort and being Italian there was food everywhere. I would find myself eating less at the dinner table and wait till everyone was asleep before I ate again. Whether I was eating because of hunger or emotionally I had no clue. I used to eat two dinners and go straight to bed. This habit continued right till I had surgery. In my junior year of High School, I weighed 192 pounds. I dieted hard and exercised to fit into my prom dress. Every second of my life I was told that I was morbidly obese.

At age twenty-three, I got involved in a car accident that led to multiple herniated discs. My weight started piling up and in six years I went from 220 pounds. to 290 pounds. This was the biggest I had ever been. My pain was getting worse and I decided not to get addicted to pain pills. My body did what my mind desired and once again, I dropped seventy pounds and felt great. That lasted a year when I got into a second car accident that set me back. It was 2016 and I weighed 350 pounds. My weight started interfering with my life. I was unable to put my shoes on or go on a roller coaster. I got engaged to be married and my grandmother asked me if I was okay being a fat bride! I started crying.

I was the bridesmaid at my best friend's wedding, and I was unable to fit into the bridesmaid dress. They had to sew two dresses together to make it fit. It was such a horrible situation, I lied to the seamstress that I had got pregnant and was still losing the weight.

I decided I need help and considered bariatric surgery. This was a matter of life and death and I needed to do something. When I found my surgeon, I followed the rules and committed myself to portion control, reading labels, and exercising. I did suffer from cravings but overcame them. I hit goal weight thirteen months after my gastric sleeve. I weigh 172 pounds. now and have kept it off over two years.

I weigh myself every day and use the Fitbit scale. Weigh-ins keep me accountable. I have explored yoga, Pilates, bike riding, and I walk my dog twice a day. My body is no longer a prisoner. I stay on my chosen path to guarantee my results. My bachelorette party was at a water park and I wore a bikini. I post before and after pictures on social media which also keeps me accountable. I love my new body and plan on keeping it forever.

Special Thoughts

Darling, you're brilliant, and your dreams matter!
- Unknown

Passion and Process

Everybody loves a plan. Weight regain after bariatric surgery needs rules, where you build total commitment to an ideology that works.

I did set out to empower the readers of this book, but realized that you do not always want to be empowered, you want to be guided and told exactly what to do to lose weight regained after surgery.

Clearly your toolbox is missing some additional tools.

My guidance serves as a framework for solving your problems, building new skills, and recognizing your triggers.

Two big hang-ups we all face when it comes to making things happen: Passion and Process. We've got to set goals that we're passionate about *(not goals that look shiny or fancy to others!)* and we've got to choose a process that excites us and plays to our strengths.

Let's make them happen now with gorgeous tools and resources for setting goals, with making plans, prioritizing what matters most, crushing projects, and habits like nobody's business, and living a beautiful, brilliant, intentional life.

This book's unique goal setting system helps you to transform your dreams into goals, and then breaks those goals down into manageable steps you'll act on every single day.

You'll be inspired and motivated as you look back on each week, remembering all the beautiful moments and all the reasons you will be thankful for. You'll be encouraged as you track the progress you've made towards your goals and review how you moved past the hard or stressful parts of your week.

Reflecting on how you've overcome a struggle will help you move forward, confidently making steady progress on your goals.

Then you'll look ahead to the next week, prioritizing your to-do list for your health and an exciting bariatric life.

***

Bariatric To-Do List
Preoperative phase
- Prepare the right way for surgery and stay motivated thereafter.
- Map out items needed during the pre-operative phase and develop skills to help rid yourself of carbohydrate cravings.
- Write out a daily meal plan with detailed timelines, purchase effective food products and stay focused.

Post-operative phase
- Develop accountability as a valuable tool.
- See your goals to completion.
- Make lifestyle changes that last.
- Create solid strategies to maintain lifelong success.

***

Life Balance Matrix

Figure Seventy-Five

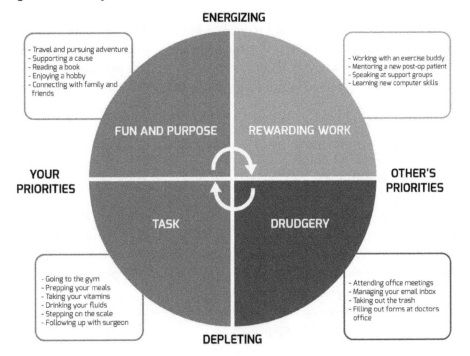

After bariatric surgery, you invariably find your life balance out of whack. Your life is so full that you just don't seem to find the time for stuff that makes you happy and fulfilled. How do you prioritize stuff that can pull your life back into balance?

The **bariatric balance matrix** is made up of an impetus axis where you get stimulated for your own priorities and other people's priorities. The energy axis is where you engage in activities that either energizes you or depletes you.

Ask yourself the following questions?

- Does this activity get me closer to something that matters to me?
- Does this activity align with my goals, values, and purpose?
- What intrinsic rewards do I get from this activity?
- Do I feel energetic after completing this activity?
- How often am I getting bored or tired by this activity?
- If I had a choice, would I do this activity for the fun of it?

Drudgery is what drains us the most. In addition to depleting your energy, it prioritizes other's needs over ours. Keep an eye on this quadrant, try to offload some of the activities, and counterbalance them by spending more time in the "Fun and Purpose" quadrant. Some examples are:

- Attending office meetings.
- Managing your email inbox.
- Taking out the trash.
- Filling out forms at doctor's office.

Tasks matter to you but still end up draining you. Keeping your annual bariatric follow-up appointment might not be the highlight of your day, but it is a relief when you complete that task. Complete tasks as efficiently as possible and combine them with fun and purpose. Get it done but do not let it take over your life. Some examples are:

- Going to the gym.
- Prepping your meals.
- Taking your vitamins.
- Drinking your fluids.
- Stepping on the scale.
- Following up with surgeon.

Rewards: Your priorities start feeling more energized. Even though the rewards might be extrinsic, you do get something like an energy boost out of it. This is a good quadrant to hang out in, but keep in mind you are still spending your energy focusing on other people's needs. Some examples are:

- Working with an exercise buddy.
- Mentoring a new post op patient.

- Speaking at support groups.
- Learning new computer skills for work.

Fun and Purpose: This is the sweet spot which matters to you the most. It boosts your core flow and makes you fall in love with life. It is a magical place to be in. if you feel your life is out of balance after bariatric surgery, it's because you don't have a lot going on in this department. Some examples are:

- Travel and pursuing adventure.
- Supporting a cause.
- Reading a book.
- Enjoying a hobby.
- Connecting with family and friends.

Plot out your activities and answer the following questions?

Of all the things you would like to do, what is calling your name out loud?

If you magically had a few hours a week to dedicate to an activity, what would you choose to devote your time to?

If time and money were not an obstacle, what would you find yourself doing in the fun and purpose quadrant?

Make room for them in your schedule by:

- Quitting something else that is not as important to you for the time being
- Delegating or offloading anything you possibly can from the *drudgery* and *task* quadrants
- Starting off by doing the tiniest version of it. Small steps build into bigger goals.

Balance your bariatric life by staying meaningful and satisfied with regular opportunities to refuel and a dash of taking out the trash.

***

Methods to Maintain Weight Loss Accountability
Measure Yourself by Weight and by Inches
Patients prefer to weigh themselves and get disheartened when the scale refuses to cooperate. Measuring your waist, hips, and arms once a week is also imperative to track the weight loss journey. This will verify commitment, maintain accountability, and deliver measurable success.

Follow Up
Keeping consultant appointments and check-ins is a biggie! This warrants accountability and nudges you toward your weight loss goals.

Bet on It
Though I am not advocating gambling, setting up some sort of stakes with a friend

who wants to lose weight is good motivation to reach your goals. Set a time frame and agree on a nonfood reward like gift cards, special outings, or tickets to an upcoming event.

***

Habits

Step one: What are your unhealthy habits?

The first step is to be aware of all your habits that are causing weight to regain after the honey moon period. Write down a list.

Did you write down any of the below?

- Drinking soda or carbonation.
- Skipping meals.
- Grazing and snacking.
- Drinking with your meals.
- Mindless eating.
- Carbohydrate addiction.
- Drinking your calories.
- Craving.
- Too lazy to exercise.
- Excessive alcohol intake.
- Believing tomorrow will be different.
- Not getting enough sleep.
- Stress.
- Not returning for post-operative appointments.
- Eating out every day.
- Smoking.
- Not drinking enough fluids.
- Not taking vitamins.
- No time to prep.

All the above thoughts and behaviors sabotage your weight loss and distract you from your goals. Every time you make one of the above choices, rather than thinking, "It's only a moment of weakness", overcome it, and keep moving along.

Step two: Pick a habit.

Identifying self-sabotaging patterns is half the battle. Pick a few of the above habits and track how many times you keep repeating it. How long you track it for depends on how frequently you indulge in that behavior. For instance, if you drink a lot of soda each day, run your tally for one day. On the other hand, if you overeat once a week rather than every day, you could tally that habit for a week.

Once you total up your tallies, it will give you a rough estimate of how often you engage in sabotaging behavior.

Step three: Break the habit

Start working on cutting the habit back by one each week. Work with your body and be gentle with it, without shocking it. In this manner, the change will last longer. For instance, if you eat dessert after dinner six times a week, cut it back by one each week. If you drink with your meals four times a day, aim for three times a day for a week and cut it back again by one the next week.

Track your progress on your phone. Once you have managed to improve on that habit pick the next one on the list.

Habits are hard to break. Here is how to troubleshoot them when you run into a wall:

- Do not rush the change but do it gradually to make it long lasting.
- Get over the initial bump and plan activities ahead of time to prevent urges from overtaking you.
- Keep in mind, you just cut back by one time every week.
- It will get easier after the first time.
- If you have trouble cutting back, give yourself time to change. Plateauing is part of any process.
- Do not find yourself falling into an ingrained habit. Catch yourself before it is too late.
- You might find yourself taking two steps forward and one step backwards. Keep moving forward.
- Most of the above habits are interlinked. Every positive or negative step has a domino effect. For instance, lack of sleep can lead to stress.
- Do not take the all or nothing approach. It takes weeks or months to build long lasting habits.

There is a magical zone of long-term success. You want to set an upper limit for any habit or goal you want to accomplish (Major, P, et al 2015,1703-17710). For example:

- I want to lose at least five pounds this month, but not more than ten pounds.
- I want to do ten pushups before my morning shower but not more than fifteen pushups.
- I want to meditate for ten minutes after I brew my morning coffee but not more than twenty minutes.

The lower limit is the minimum threshold you want to hit. You will push yourself for weight loss progress but not to such an extent that it is a miracle that never happens (A) or that it burns you out and becomes unsustainable (B). Upper limits make it easier for you to consistently show up. **The window between (A) and (B) on the graph is the zone of long-term success.**

Figure Seventy-Six

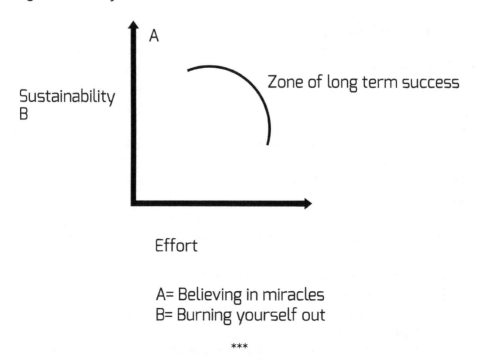

A= Believing in miracles
B= Burning yourself out

***

Do's and Don'ts on Your Bariatric Journey

DO celebrate every pound you lose. That pound is gone from your body and it is worth a pat on the back.

DON'T compare your success and failures with others. Every body's journey is their own. Comparing will only leave you disappointed.

DO keep one set of your preoperative clothes around. Make sure to try them on when you are having a down moment. This will create positivity during the roller-coaster of a ride.

DON'T save any more than one set of preoperative clothes. Give them away at a clothing swap or donate them.

DO keep a preoperative picture close by so you can look at it and compare yourself. Celebrate your loss.

DON'T believe the myth that surgery will keep it off forever. That is your individual responsibility.

DO take measurements of yourself often and keep track of inches you lose when the scale starts acting stubborn.

DON'T let the scale define you. Fluctuations and stalls happen during your journey. Patience is the key here.

DO challenge yourself to stay motivated and always willing to go further than you ever thought you would.

DON'T believe the myth that your tool has an expiration date. Though you lose the most during the first year, if you keep up with the healthy eating and fitness routines you will continue to lose weight.

DO keep a list of non-scale victories (NSV) to reflect on when times get hard. Are you able to tie your shoelaces? Are you able to take a plane ride without asking for an extension belt?

DON'T be afraid to change things that are not working. If you are on a long stall, change your eating patterns and activity around.

***

Lose-Your-Regain Activity # fifteen: Laugh More and Stress Less

Duration: Five minutes

A good laugh increases the levels of your feel-good endorphins in your brain. Make laughter a part of your life to relax your tense muscles. Seek out something funny to improve your immune system, relieve your pain and better cope with stressful situations.

How to complete the activity:

- Bookmark a few funny things on your phone or computer. It could be a funny podcast, videos of cats in sticky situations, your favorite comedian on YouTube. Chuckle by reading a book of hilarious stories.
- For the next five days, if you feel stressed, spend five minutes listening, watching, or reading something hilarious. Cracking up will make you feel calmer and more relaxed instantly.

https://go.omadahealth.com

(Health, Omada. "The Omada Program.")

***

Meet Edwin who after years of dieting and deprivation, put an end to the rebellion and follows his new weight loss surgery lifestyle. Read about how he uses gratitude to get out of discouragement. Write down five things you are grateful for.

Figure Seventy-Seven *(see next page)*

Edwin: I have been overweight my whole life, well, maybe not my whole life, if I can remember. There are pictures of me from my early childhood looking like a "normal" child, but from the time that I was about eight or nine I was the chubby kid. I was the kid that had to wear what was called "Husky" sizes at the time, who even from an early age had to go with my mom to stores to get suits and "dressy" clothes.

From a husky kid to a heavy teen to an adult who had to shop only in Big and Tall stores, not even stores with Big and Tall sections, but stores that specialized in clothing for big people.

I can't tell you when I finally decided I needed to change my life. I tried Weight Watchers, which was success-

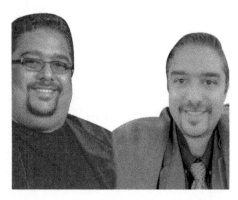

ful, until it wasn't. Atkins, South Beach, Sugar Free, Soups, Slim Fast, prepackaged meals, premade shakes, pills, they all worked at first and then I would gain it all back.

I needed to do something drastic. I have a daughter who I want to see graduate from College. I want to walk her down the aisle, and more than that, I knew all the things that my weight had stolen from us – being able to dance more than one song, ride roller coasters, and so on.

I have a wife. The plan is to be eighty-years-old and hold hands in the park. My weight was putting that at risk.

And beyond that I was slowly becoming less and less mobile. I was always the guy who was told "was so agile for your size" or "so flexible for your size" or "could really move for your size," but, as I got older that was becoming less and less the case. My knees were shot. My back had gotten messed up in a car accident. I couldn't fit in an airplane seat. I needed an extender in my car to wear my seatbelt. Desperate times called for desperate measures.

That was when I returned to New York and finally had an insurance plan that would cover weight loss surgery. When I sought Bariatric surgery, I was stunned when I stood on the scale and saw 488 pounds. It was clear to me that gastric sleeve was the way to go.

In the two years since bariatric surgery, I have lost 145 pounds.

Am I anywhere near my goal yet?

No.

Have I had setbacks?

Yes.

Do I have it all figured out?

No.

Do I have a long way to go?

Yes.

Was Gastric sleeve surgery the instant magic easy solution people think it is?

No.

Was it an AMAZING tool that helped get me started on the road to health and recovery?

Yes.

I have had to be make the decision that I was going to do it. That was all. The surgery was a way to reboot my system, but after that it was up to me to stay on track and not allow old habits to creep back in and reverse the progress that I had made. It has required discipline. It has required that I focus on what was important. I have had to learn to eat to live, not live to eat.

I keep track of what I am eating. I set limits and boundaries and make decisions based on those things. I had to think about cakes and cookies the way an alcoholic does alcohol. Have I slowly been able to have one cookie, or one slice? Yes. But I had to recreate my relationship with food. And when I mess up, which I do, I need to reboot.

I have had to occasionally go back to protein shakes for a day or two to remind myself of how my tool works. I have had to change my habits. I eat off salad plates instead of dinner plates. I pay attention to portions. I keep track of how many carbs I eat daily.

I have not become an obsessive calorie and carb counter. I have made it a point to do things to get more mobile. I park far away from the place where I am going, so that I must walk farther. I make it a point to walk during my lunch break. I go for walks with my wife. And then I joined a gym.

Am I a crazy gym head? No. But I use the treadmill on rainy days when I can't go for a walk. I go swimming in the pool. I make a conscious decision to be mobile and active. I am not going to lie and say, "I love exercise now!!" But I don't hate it anymore, and I have truly learned that the benefits are huge.

Resources

Cottage Cheese Pouch Test

If you have regained weight after bariatric surgery, this four-step pouch test will make you aware if the "tool" is still intact and effective in restricting food intake. Stay away from food and fluids for sixty-minutes before the pouch test. Test the effectiveness of your pouch during the first meal of the day.

Figure Seventy-Eight

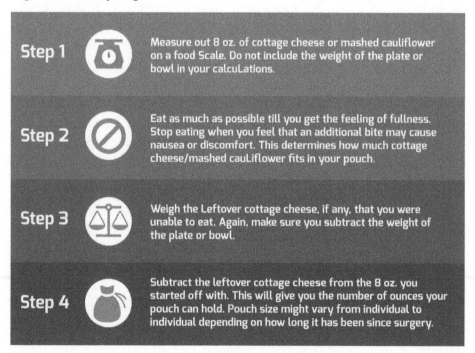

Step 1 Measure out 8 oz. of cottage cheese or mashed cauliflower on a food Scale. Do not include the weight of the plate or bowl in your calcuLations.

Step 2 Eat as much as possible till you get the feeling of fullness. Stop eating when you feel that an additional bite may cause nausea or discomfort. This determines how much cottage cheese/mashed cauLiflower fits in your pouch.

Step 3 Weigh the Leftover cottage cheese, if any, that you were unable to eat. Again, make sure you subtract the weight of the plate or bowl.

Step 4 Subtract the leftover cottage cheese from the 8 oz. you started off with. This will give you the number of ounces your pouch can hold. Pouch size might vary from individual to individual depending on how long it has been since surgery.

Repeat these steps every three to four months to see how your pouch size increases with time.

***

Figure Seventy-Nine

EGGS AND BELL PEPPERS:
While eggs are a great source of protein and contain choline to boost your metabolism bell peppers offer crunch and vitamin C to ward off cortisol.

OATMEAL AND BERRIES:
A great breakfast option that contributes insoluble fiber from the oatmeal and polyphenols from the berries to help combat fat storage.

TUNA AND GINGER
Pair either a tuna roll or tuna sashimi with pickled ginger to reduce bloat - causing inflammation and provide omega - 3 fatty acids.

YOGURT AND CINNAMON:
Improve insulin sensitivity by sprinkling cinnamon on vitamin D fortified yogurt.

PUMPKIN SEEDS AND GREENS
Sprinkle an ounce of protein packed pumpkin seeds on your salads for a satisfying lunch.

WALNUTS AND RASPBERRIES:
Pair healthy fat like walnuts with these fiber - packed ruby jewels to get a pick me up 3 pm snack.

BANANA AND NUT BUTTER:
Stay full longer with nut butters and a healthy source of carbohydrates

CHICK PEAS AND OLIVE OIL:
Roast this superfood that is high in fiber and increase satiety by combining it with extra virgin olive oil (EVOO).

HUMMUS AND CARROTS:
Look for single serving containers of this high fiber, healthy fat snack while reaping it's benefits on the go.

APPLES AND PEANUT BUTTER:
Smear all-natural peanut butter on crunchy slices of apples to stay satiated till your next meal.

GREEN TEA AND MINT:
Steep some sprigs of mint leaves in a cup of tea after dinner and squash any after dinner cravings.

CUCUMBER SLICES AND EGG SALAD:
Hydrate yourself with cucumber slices topped with egg salad for a crunchy high protein shack.

***

Figure Eighty

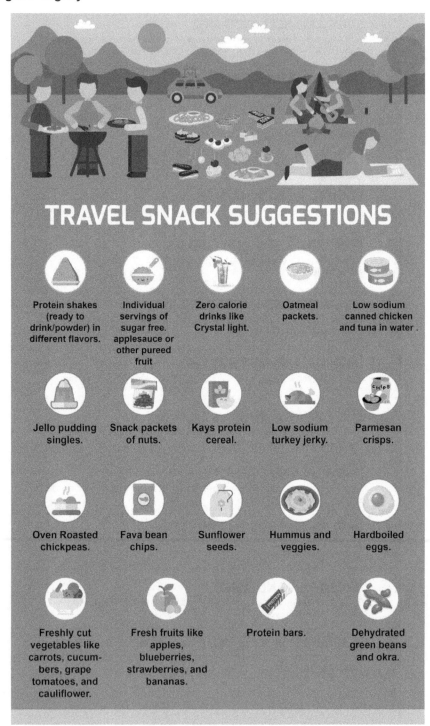

Figure Eighty-One

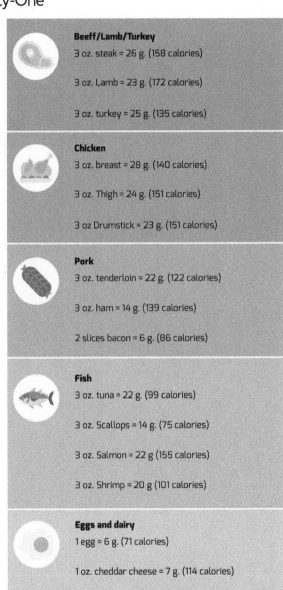

Beeff/Lamb/Turkey

3 oz. steak = 26 g. (158 calories)

3 oz. Lamb = 23 g. (172 calories)

3 oz. turkey = 25 g. (135 calories)

Chicken

3 oz. breast = 28 g. (140 calories)

3 oz. Thigh = 24 g. (151 calories)

3 oz Drumstick = 23 g. (151 calories)

Pork

3 oz. tenderloin = 22 g. (122 calories)

3 oz. ham = 14 g. (139 calories)

2 slices bacon = 6 g. (86 calories)

Fish

3 oz. tuna = 22 g. (99 calories)

3 oz. Scallops = 14 g. (75 calories)

3 oz. Salmon = 22 g (155 calories)

3 oz. Shrimp = 20 g (101 calories)

Eggs and dairy

1 egg = 6 g. (71 calories)

1 oz. cheddar cheese = 7 g. (114 calories)

1 cup skim milk = 8 g. (86 calories)

1 cup yogurt (plain) = 11 g. (100 calories)

6 oz. Greek yogurt = 18 g. (100 calories)

Source: 2013 Today's Dietitian

***

Figure Eighty-Two

FOOD	SERVING	PROTEIN (g)
Cooked black beans	1/2 cup	8
Cooked lentils	1/2 cup	9
Cooked Pinto beans	1/2 cup	8
Regular Tofu	4 ounces	10
Cooked split peas	1/2 cup	8
Cooked white beans	1/2 cup	8
Cooked chickpeas	1/2 cup	8
Cooked kidney beans	1/2 cup	8
Cooked Fava beans	1/2 cup	7
Almonds	1 ounce	6
Brazil nuts	1 ounce (6-8 nuts)	4
Cashews	1 ounce (18 nuts)	4
Hazelnuts	1 ounce (21 nuts)	4
Walnuts	1 ounce (14 halves)	4
Macademia nuts	1 ounce (10-12 nuts)	2
Peanuts	1 ounce (25 nuts)	7
Peanut butter	2 T	8
Flaxseeds	1 ounce (3 T)	5
Chia seeds	1 ounce (2 1/2T)	4
Hemp seeds	1 ounce (3 T)	9
Pine nuts	1 ounce (3 T)	4
Pistachios	1 ounce (3 1/2 T)	6
Sunflower seeds	1 ounce (3 1/2 T)	5

***

Figure Eighty-Three

FRUIT	QUANTITY	CARB CONTENT
RASPBERRIES	1/2 CUP	3 GRAMS
STRAWBERRIES	1/2 CUP	6 GRAMS
BLACKBERRIES	1/2 CUP	4 GRAMS
BLUEBERRIES	1/2 CUP	6 GRAMS
PLUM	1 MEDIUM	6 GRAMS
MANDARIN	1 MEDIUM	7 GRAMS
KIWI	1 MEDIUM	8 GRAMS
CHERRIES	1/2 CUP	9 GRAMS
CANTALOUPE	1 CUP	11 GRAMS
PEACH	1 MEDIUM	13 GRAMS

Credit: (Gundry, 2017)

Choose one from **list A** and one from **list B** for a balanced bariatric friendly snack.

Figure Eighty-Four

BARIATRIC FRIENDLY SNACKS

Choose one from list A and one from list B for a balanced friendly snack.

LIST A
Almonds
Walnuts
Pumpkin seeds
Sunflower seeds
Hummus
Almond butter
Peanut butter
Egg salad
String cheese
Feta cheese
Hard-boiled egg
Chicken salad
Salmon salad
Toasted sweet potato slice
Yogurt
Ricotta cheese
Cottage cheese
Sliced cheese
Shrimp
Goat cheese
Sliced mozzarella

LIST B
Sliced tomato
Parmesan crisps
Edamame
Low sodium cold cuts
Baby carrots
Olives
Grapes
Cucumber slices
Water melon
Cauliflower florets
Pear
Apple
Strawberries
Pomegranate seeds
Blueberries
Guacamole
Applesauce
Fresh cold cuts
Cocktail sauce
Jicama
Salsa

Bariatric Kitchen Tools

- As an alternative to plastic lunch bags, lunch skins are food safe reusable, washable bags made from heat tolerant fabric and can safely hold anything from carrot sticks to apple slices to hot sandwiches. www.lunchskins.com
- Ditch plastic wrap for Bee's Wrap. Made of cotton muslin dipped in beeswax, it is reusable and molds with the warmth of your hands. www.bees-wrap.com
- Designed after the Japanese bento boxes that hold dishes in separate compartments. Stainless steel, these lunch boxes are perfect for the bariatric adult who does not like his/her foods comingled. www.planetbox.com
- Silicone encased shatter resistant glass food storage containers can be used in freezers and ovens. www.fregoliving.com
- A slow cooker that is fitted with an organic clay pot to prevent plastic or leached chemicals to touch the food. www.vitaclaychef.com
- Glass water bottles with a silicone sleeve sidestep the issue of leached chemicals. The wide mouth makes it easy to add ice cubes and tea bags, making it easy to wash. www.lifefactory.com
- Perfect water bottle equipped with a self-sealing side pocket to hold your keys, cash and cards. www.gocontigo.com
- When tap water is all that is available, filter it yourself with this bisphenol A (BPA) free container that contains a replaceable charcoal filter. It reduces chlorine, adds minerals, and cleans up the taste. Filters last up to six months. www.blackblum.com
- A water bottle for a cyclist. Stainless steel BPA free bottle, it unscrews at both ends for easy cleaning. www.cleanbottle.com
- The GoStak compartments screw together so you can bring your vitamins, protein powder, and backup snacks all together for your overnight trips. www.blenderbottle.com
- This handy stacking tiffin box carries an entire meal with accompanying side dishes to work. www.mightynest.com
- Enjoy hot lunches with this stainless steel airtight thermos pot that keeps contents warm for up to six hours. A magnetic spoon attaches itself to the side of the cup. www.blackblum.com
- Airtight coverings are created with nontoxic materials like hemp, beeswax, jojoba oil to keep food fresh and safe. Hand washable in cold water. www.abeego.ca
- Ice cream pop molds are stackable and come with lids to protect the frozen dessert. www.lekueusa.com

- Three-blade hand held spiralizer is BPA free and ribbon cuts fresh veggies. www.oxo.com

From the Bariatric Pantry

- Never run out of hummus. This mix comes in a box that you stir up with a little water and olive oil. www.fantasticfoods.com
- Plant based protein shakes that pack easily and mix with water. Comes in different flavors. www.myvega.com
- Green tea has a grassy flavor and is rich in antioxidants. www.rishi-tea.com
- Ginger kombucha soothes an upset stomach, and helps to rebuild gut bacteria. www.synergydrinks.com
- Barbeque pork jerky packs nine grams of protein for each one ounce serving. www.kravejerky.com
- *Chobani* smoked onion and parmesan Meze dip offers three grams of protein and twenty five calories for every two-tablespoon serving. www.freshdirect.com
- Chia pods give you six grams of fiber in every six-oz. cup. Made up of chia seeds, water, vanilla bean, banana puree and coconut milk.
- Organic seaweed snacks are crunchy and a good source of vitamin C. An entire five-gram package has only twenty five calories. www.gimmehealth.com
- Pair pomegranate seeds with low fat plain yogurt to harness loads of cancer fighting polyphenols. A hundred - calorie cup has fresh pomegranate seeds as its only ingredients. Available at your local supermarket.
- Hippeas chick pea puffs are addictive, crunchy, and airy. Made from non-GMO chick peas, a one ounce bag contributes 130 calories, five grams of fat, three grams of fiber and four grams of protein. Available at your local grocery store.
- Crunchy kale offers impressive amounts of vitamins A and C. Each two ounce bag offers eighty calories, six grams of fat, two grams of fiber and three grams of protein. www.bradsplantbased.com
- Roasted chickpeas have a good amount of protein to keep you satiated. One and quarter ounce serving offers 130 calories, four grams of fat, five grams of fiber and six grams of protein. At local Wholefoods stores.
- "Made in Nature" veggie pops are made from organic kale, chickpeas, cauliflower, and bell peppers. A one and quarter ounce serving offers 140 calories, eight grams of fat, four grams of fiber and eight grams of protein. Available on amazon.
- "From the ground, up" Cauliflower pretzels satisfy your cravings and are made from cauliflower. A four and a half ounce bag offers 110 calories,

one and half grams of fat, three grams of fiber, and one gram of protein. www.jet.com

- "Wilde" chicken chips are made with chicken breasts, tapioca flour, and coconut oil. Offers more protein than usual. A two and half ounce bag has 170 calories, ten grams of fat, and seven grams of protein. www.barefoot-provisions.com
- Rhythm Superfoods Organic carrot sticks are made from nothing but dehydrated carrots. A 1.4 oz. bag offers 140 calories, one and half grams of fat, eleven grams of fiber, and three grams of protein. www.thrivemarket.com
- Simple Mills almond flour crackers are gluten free and hefty enough to hold your cheeses and dips. A four and quarter ounce box offers 150 calories, eight grams of fat, two grams of fiber, and three grams of protein. www.simplemills.com
- Roth Snack Cheese consists of gouda, cheddar, or mozzarella rounds at seventy calories a pop along with five grams of fat and five grams of protein. www.rothcheese.com
- Mushroom jerky delivers 45% of your daily vitamin D needs and 21% of fiber. A 2.2 oz. bag offers 110 calories, seven grams of fat, six grams of fiber, and one gram of protein. www.mushroomjerky.com
- Chicken jerky is made with antibiotic free chicken for a leaner bite. The siracha flavor is addictive. A 2.25 oz. bag offers seventy calories, one and half grams of fat, and ten grams of protein. www.epicbar.com
- Vanilla almond butter is a portable packet and can be spread on apples or nuts. A 1.13 oz. pouch offers 190 calories, fifteen grams of fat, two grams of fiber, and nine grams of protein. www.target.com
- Gaea Cauliflower snack has pickled cauliflower and is a savory, tangy treat. A 2.8 oz. pack offers ten calories, zero grams of fat, less than one gram of protein. www.gaeaolive.com
- Smash mallow crispy treats are made from all natural ingredients and has a cinnamon churro flavor. A 1.15 oz. bag offers 130 calories, three and half grams of fat and two grams of protein. www.smashmallow.com
- Faba Butter is a dairy free butter made from coconut cream and aquafaba (the thick water that chickpeas float in within a can). Spread it on apples and veggies and even cook with it. Available at all Eatalys nationwide.
- Veggies that are washed and flash frozen soon after being harvested, are then dolled up with parmesan cheese or olive oil. www.lisasorganics.com
- Gluten and dairy free soup concoctions available in six ounce containers. Carrot ginger soup, zucchini soup, red lentil veggie soup, and tomato soup are some of the offerings. www.cooksf.com

- Cheesy Kale chips are savory, crunchy, and wholesome. www.justpurefoods.com
- Gourmet Teas that can be poured over ice come in various flavors like Mango Ceylon with vanilla and Moroccan Mint Green. www.choiceorganictea.com
- Kitchen Basics unsalted chicken stock is the best tasting, unsalted cooking stock out there. Available at your local food stores.
- Quick oats come in individual sachets with no added salt or sugar. www.naturespath.com

Dinner at Your Door Step

CAUTION: The following are just suggestions and may not be bariatric friendly regarding calories, carb content, and protein content. Please look at them further before deciding to take this route.

- **HelloFresh** has been around since 2012 and offers chef - curated recipes that include meat, fish and vegetarian meal kits. It arrives in insulated boxes, and is delivered both nationwide and internationally. www.hellofresh.com
- **Blue Apron** is a subscription-based model that offers vegetarian, pescetarian, and omnivore plans. Fresh ingredients and recipes are shipped nationwide. www.blueapron.com
- **Plated** focuses on fresh ingredients and globally inspired recipes like the salmon poke bowl, beef tacos, and chicken marsala. www.plated.com
- **Terra's Kitchen** offers meal types for vegetarians, gluten free meals, vegans etc. Turkey spinach balls and pecan- crusted tilapia are some of the meals. Ships nationwide. www.terraskitchen.com
- **Martha and Mailey Spoon** makes cooking easy on busy week nights while supporting local farmers. Recipe cards include smart cooking techniques www.marleyspoon.com
- **Peachdish** is all about the south. Think butternut squash and three-bean chili. Ships nationwide. www.peachdish.com
- **Green Chef** offers chef -developed recipes that take less than forty five minutes to cook. Ninety-five percent of its ingredients are organic and can be tracked from supplier to dinner table. https://greenchef.com/home

Outdoor Essentials

- Hand welded steel rings can be slung over a swing set or sturdy tree for the perfect workout at the park or in your own backyard. www.roguefitness.com
- Take your workout anywhere with this set of five resistance bands ranging from two to seventy five pounds. Weighing only thirty two ounces, it fits neatly into your backpack. Perfect for road warriors. www.blackmountainproducts.com

- This nubby rubber acuball applies pressure to tight muscles including the spine. Heat it in the microwave for extra comfort. www.acuball.com
- A jump rope is a portable fitness tool that raises your heart rate and improves coordination. Rubber grips and nylon cord resists any twisting. www.humanxgear.com
- Have a personal golf coach with a Swing byte analyzer where a sensor attaches to your golf club and delivers a 3D image of your swing to an app. www.swingbyte.com
- Kettle bells offer a challenging combo of cardio and strength workouts. www.lifelinefitness.com
- Yoga socks keep your feet covered while leaving your toes free to grip the floor. www.toesox.com
- Hula hoop workouts loosen your hips and give you a vigorous core workout. It is collapsible and serves as a great travel companion. www.canyonhoops.com
- A terrific online resource called "Do yoga with me" has free light stretching/ yoga classes to choose from. www.doyogawithme.com

Figure Eighty-Five

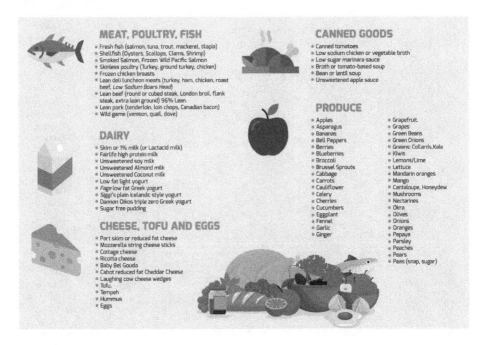

MEAT, POULTRY, FISH
- Fresh fish (salmon, tuna, trout, mackerel, tilapia)
- Shellfish (Oysters, Scallops, Clams, Shrimp)
- Smoked Salmon, Frozen Wild Pacific Salmon
- Skinless poultry (Turkey, ground turkey, chicken)
- Frozen chicken breasts
- Lean deli luncheon meats (turkey, ham, chicken, roast beef, *Low Sodium Boars Head*)
- Lean beef (round or cubed steak, London broil, flank steak, extra lean ground) 96% Lean.
- Lean pork (tenderloin, loin chops, Canadian bacon)
- Wild game (venison, quail, dove)

DAIRY
- Skim or 1% milk (or Lactacid milk)
- Fairlife high protein milk
- Unsweetened soy milk
- Unsweetened Almond milk
- Unsweetened Coconut milk
- Low fat light yogurt
- Fage low fat Greek yogurt
- Siggi's plain Icelandic style yogurt
- Dannon Oikos triple zero Greek yogurt
- Sugar free pudding

CHEESE, TOFU AND EGGS
- Part skim or reduced fat cheese
- Mozzarella string cheese sticks
- Cottage cheese
- Ricotta cheese
- Baby Bel Gouda
- Cabot reduced fat Cheddar Cheese
- Laughing cow cheese wedges
- Tofu.
- Tempeh
- Hummus
- Eggs

CANNED GOODS
- Canned tomatoes
- Low sodium chicken or vegetable broth
- Low sugar marinara sauce
- Broth or tomato-based soup
- Bean or lentil soup
- Unsweetened apple sauce

PRODUCE
- Apples
- Asparagus
- Bananas
- Bell Peppers
- Berries
- Blueberries
- Broccoli
- Brussel Sprouts
- Cabbage
- Carrots
- Cauliflower
- Celery
- Cherries
- Cucumbers
- Eggplant
- Fennel
- Garlic
- Ginger
- Grapefruit.
- Grapes
- Green Beans
- Green Onions
- Greens: Collards, Kale
- Kiwis
- Lemons/Lime
- Lettuce
- Mandarin oranges
- Mango
- Cantaloupe, Honeydew
- Mushrooms
- Nectarines
- Okra
- Olives
- Onions
- Oranges
- Papaya
- Parsley
- Peaches
- Pears
- Peas (snap, sugar)

Figure Eighty-Six

	Breakfast	Snack	Lunch	Snack	Dinner
Monday	3 oz. raspberry Overnight Oats.	4 baby carrots and 1 Tbsp. almond butter.	3 oz. Chicken sausage and Broccoli.	1 Hard-boiled egg and sliced cucumbers.	3 oz. Chicken or fish tacos in lettuce wraps.
Tuesday	1 cup Greek yogurt with raspberries and almonds.	1 small apple and 1 Tbsp. peanut butter.	1 Salmon cake with hummus.	3 oz. Cottage cheese and peaches.	1 stuffed Portobello mushroom pizza with cheese and tomato sauce.
Wednesday	1 Meatless breakfast patty with 1 egg.	Skillet popped lentils.	3 oz. Turkey chili.	Spinach Quinoa patties.	1 zucchini boat with seasoned chopped meat.
Thursday	3 oz. guacamole stuffed eggs.	Banana chia pudding.	3 oz. tuna salad.	Black bean hummus with carrot sticks.	3 oz. Cauliflower pizza topped with veggies and cheese.
Friday	1 egg and cheese omelet.	Spinach quinoa patties.	Avocado chicken salad.	3 oz. ricotta cheese and 1/2 pear.	1 stuffed red pepper with chopped turkey, and cauliflower rice.
Saturday	Almond flour pancakes with berries.	Almond crusted salmon sticks.	3 oz. Chickpea. salad.	3 oz. watermelon with a sprinkling of feta cheese.	Turkey meatballs with asparagus tips.
Sunday	3 oz. of a breakfast bowl (eggs.sweet potatoes, nuts, quinoa).	3 oz. Greek yogurt.	1 falafel waffle topped with veggies.	10 nuts and a cheese stick.	3 oz. of stir fry shrimp and cauliflower rice.

Figure Eighty-Seven

BARIATRIC BREAKFAST WINNERS

YOGURT WITH BERRIES AND SEEDS
3-4 Ounces Plain Greek yogurt + berries + pumpkin/chia/flax seeds

SMOKED SALMON AND EGG STUFFED AVOCADOS
1 egg + 2 Ounces smoked salmon +1/2 avocado +Dill +Chili flakes +Spices

SPINACH TOMATO SCRAMBLE
2 Eggs + Spinach +Cherry Tomatoes

NUT BUTTER AND BERRY YOGURT
3-4 ounces Greek Yogurt +1 tsp Nut butter +berries

SOUTHWESTERN TOFU SCRAMBLE
3-4 ounces Tofu +veggies +Herbs

GREENS AND GARLIC FRITTATA
2 Eggs +Greens +Garlic +Cheese

SPINACH AND EGG WHITE OMELET
1 Egg +Spinach +Cheese

ZUCCHINI WAFFLES
2 Eggs + Zucchini + Onions + Cheese

AVOCADO BASIL YOGURT PARFAIT
3-4 ounces Greek Yogurt +1/2 Avocado +Basil

CHEESY VEGGIE EGG MUFFINS
2 Eggs + Cheese + Veggies

CINNAMON PEAR TOFU SMOOTHIE
3-4 ounces Silken Tofu +Pears +Unsweetened
almond milk +Flaxseed meal

Figure Eighty -Eight

BARIATRIC LUNCH WINNERS

PAN FRIED TILAPIA WITH MUSHROOMS
3 ounces Tilapia +Porcini mushrooms +lemon + scallions

TURKEY CHILI
3 ounces Ground turkey +spices + salsa

TOFU BENTO BOWL
3 ounces' tofu + 2 ounces' yogurt +veggies +lemon
+ginger +chili garlic sauce + sesame seeds

TUNA SALAD IN AVOCADO SHELL
3 ounces' tuna salad +1/2 avocado +lemon

CAULIFLOWER CHEDDAR SOUP
3 ounces Cheddar Cheese +Cauliflower +Bell Pepper +Broth

BLACK BEAN QUINOA BURGERS
3 ounces of black beans +2 ounces of quinoa
+shallot +garlic +egg white +lime

SEITAN(WHEAT GLUTEN) STIR FRY
3 ounces of seitan + onion +garlic + ginger +
sesame seeds + broccoli +bell pepper

CHICKEN STUFFED BELL PEPPERS
3 ounces of chopped chicken +bell pepper
+cauliflower rice + grated cheese

TZATZIKI CHICKEN SALAD
3 ounces' chicken +3 ounces plain yogurt +onion
+lemon +dill +cucumber +garlic +greens

SHRIMP WITH GARLIC
3 ounces of shrimp +garlic +dried red chili +parsley

Figure Eighty-Nine

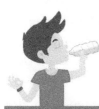

BARIATRIC DINNER WINNERS

Baked Halibut and Spinach
3 ounces' halibut +herbs +orange +spinach

Lamb Chops with Tomatoes and Olives
3-4 ounces' lamb chop +tomatoes +olives +shallots

Tofu, Spinach, and Sesame Stir Fry
3 ounces' tofu +garlic +ginger +spinach +sesame seeds -hot chilli flakes +sesame oil

Turkey Skillet Dinner
3 ounces ground turkey +zucchini +onion +tomatoes +tomato paste

Dijon Pork and Asparagus
3 ounces' pork +asparagus +tarragon +scallions +mustard

Shrimp, Tomato, and Avocado Salad
3 ounces' shrimp +avocado +cherry tomatoes +veggies +lime + Lettuce

Lemon Chicken and Cauliflower Soup
3 ounces' chicken +cauliflower +low sodium chicken broth +lemon +onion +garlic +rosemary +oilve oil

Poached Sole with Capers
3 ounces sole +capers +olives +low sodium broth +salad greens

Chicken and Vegetables
3 ounces chicken +carrots +onion +diced tomatoes +tomato paste +celery

Celebrating the Holidays Bariatric Style

Holiday Recipe Swap: Swap Old Favorites for New Ones

Though the holidays are a wonderful time to celebrate and enjoy delicious food, it does not have to mean throwing a wedge into your bariatric journey! Use this table to help swap out some of the less healthy holiday favorites for reinvented, healthier bariatric-friendly alternatives.

Figure Ninety

	OLD FAVORITE	NEW FAVORITE
HORS D'OEUVRES	SPINACH ARTICHOKE DIP	**Holiday Spinach Dip with Fresh veggies** Make a healthier version, loaded with healthy fats, veggies, and flavor, which works great hot or cold and serve with chopped raw vegetables.
	CHIPS AND DIP	**Pumpkin Hummus with Apple Chips** Loaded with fiber, this savory sweet dip works great with apple chips (make your own or buy an unsweetened version) or even fresh apple slices.
	DEVILED EGGS	**Baked Artichoke Hearts** A flavor packed vegetable-based alternative to that one bite party appetizers.
	TRADITIONAL BREADED MEATBALLS	**Crumb-less, Turkey Meatballs** This breadcrumb free version uses shredded carrot to bind together.
APPETIZERS	CAESAR SALAD	**Beet and Crumbled Goat Cheese Salad** Nutrient packed, with healthy fats and veggies.
ENTREES	HONEY BAKED HAM, PRIME RIB, WHOLE TURKEY	**Kale and Herb Stuffed Turkey Breast** A leaner cut with added vegetables for extra nutrients.
	STUFFED CABBAGE ROLLS	**Grain Free Unstuffed Cabbage Rolls** By deconstructing, this version contains no grains and a no sugar added tomato sauce, but keeps all those traditional flavors you love.
	LASAGNA PASTA	**Vegetarian Sweet Potato Lasagna** This noodle free version is a great option for a vegetarian entree, packed full of veggies without dramatically compromising your family favorite
SIDES	MASHED POTATOES, CANDIED YAMS	**Roasted Squash** Fresh, nutty flavors that let you enjoy your fall starchy vegetable without the sugar load
	GREEN BEAN CASSEROLE CANDIED CARROTS	**Brussel Sprouts with Pecans** Keep your vegetables nutrient dense with this easy roasting, and with healthy fats to boot from the pecans.

Figure Ninety-One

INITIAL STATS (FEMALE)

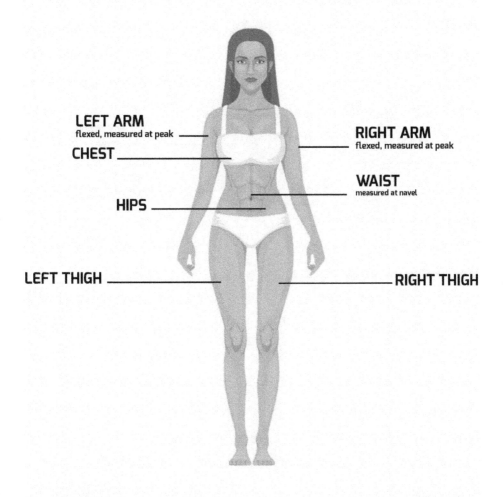

LEFT ARM
flexed, measured at peak

CHEST

RIGHT ARM
flexed, measured at peak

WAIST
measured at navel

HIPS

LEFT THIGH

RIGHT THIGH

DATE

Figure Ninety-Two

INITIAL STATS (MALE)

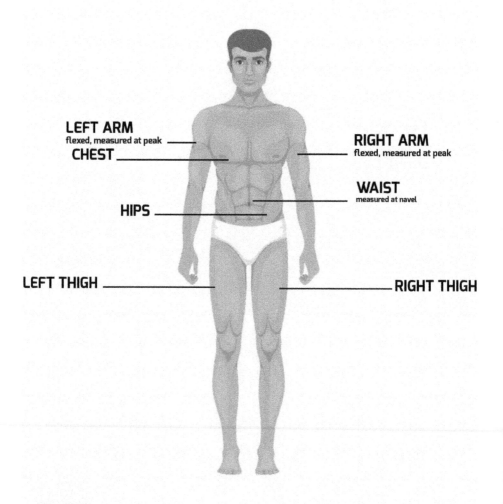

LEFT ARM
flexed, measured at peak ——

CHEST ———

RIGHT ARM
flexed, measured at peak

WAIST
measured at navel

HIPS ———

LEFT THIGH ———

RIGHT THIGH

DATE

Figure Ninety-Three

SPECIAL MENU REQUEST

The person presenting this card had a surgical procedure,
resulting in their stomach capacity being reduced.
Please allow him/her to order a smaller
half portion or make a selection from the kids/seniors menu

MANY THANKS FOR YOUR COOPERATION

Acknowledgements

I would like to acknowledge some of the most important people, all of whom in one way or the other made the process of writing this book possible.

First and foremost, I would like to thank God for giving me the gift of compassion for people and the desire to pass along knowledge with the hope that it helps and creates a positive impact in the life of bariatric patients.

I thank my parents, Shama and Taj, for the secure, loving family base you created in my life. I'm blessed to be your daughter. To my brother, Sajid for believing in all I take on. You all know that family is everything to me.

To my son and daughter – Kamran and Ayda. You are the best things I ever created! Both of you are so smart and have taught me so much. I have enjoyed watching both of you become focused, personable, and successful human beings.

For my family, who lift me up, particularly, Frank. and Patricia Riccuiti. I am so proud to be a part of our crazy family.

And especially my handsome husband Frank Riccuiti, Jr. Thank you for your love and support. You have believed in me, even when there were moments I did not.

Special thanks to Dr. Dominick Gadaleta and Dr. Larry Gellman for providing a work environment that is respectful, enriching, and rewarding. Both of you are visionaries with a commitment to excellence, and it has been an exhilarating ride. I am indebted to many professionals in the field of bariatrics, be they psychologists, dietitians, social workers, exercise physiologists, nurse practitioners, and pharmacists who have worked together for the success of the bariatric patient.

I am also thankful each day for each one of my patients for allowing me to be a part of their lives and giving back more than I can express. Each one of you is the purpose of my life.

Special credit goes to Danna Russo, Tom Nasso, Melissa Johnson, Beth Falon, Vickie Brown, Jamal Stewart, Elizabeth Nolan, Raquel Welch, Frank Montalbo, Tina Baker, Emily Belmonte, Karen Iamartino, Maria Genao and Edwin Velazquez for talking about their successes and failures during their weight loss journey.

I'm thankful for Tammy "St. Clair" for contributing toward the "Mindless Eating" section and discussing how bariatric surgery has changed her life.

Dr. Nicole Pecquex and Dr. William Richardson for their views on why patients regain weight after surgery.

Special thanks to Jel Gueco for always being there, draft after draft, helping me turn my dreams into reality and Janet Godsberg in helping me polish the manuscript.

To the Morgan James Publishing team: Special thanks to David Hancock, CEO & Founder for believing in me and my message. To my Author Relations Manager, Bonnie Rauch, thanks for making the process seamless and easy. Many more thanks to everyone else, but especially Jim Howard, Bethany Marshall, and Nickcole Watkins. Above all I want to thank my editor Todd Hunter for his patience with me in the authorship of my first book.

Thank You

Thank you for allowing me to guide you along your weight loss journey. I appreciate the time you have taken to read this book and hope it gave you the answers you are looking for along with tips and strategies to keep your weight regain off. I understand that there is a lot of information and could be overwhelming. If you would like to work with me to help you go through the various steps of "Regain be Gone" that I discuss in the book, and reach your weight loss goals faster, please reach out to me to schedule a strategy session to see if we are the right fit. Just go to www.lowkcalgal and pick a time to chat.

Thanks again and may your weight loss journey be enlightening and everlasting!

Connect with Sameera at:
Website: www.lowkcalgal.com
Email: health@lowkcalgal.com
Facebook: www.facebook.com/lowkcalgal
Instagram: @lowkcalgal

Just for You

Congratulations! You now have the plan to keep yourself free from regain. But do you know what will help you more?

A journal on overcoming cravings. This journal will walk you through step-by-step the path to take to freedom from giving in to your urges. It's NOT going to do the work for you, but it will show you precisely what you can do right now to SUBDUE THE HANKERING. This is how you're going to stay in charge during your life - long weight loss journey

If you are ready to take control of your cravings once and for all..........then visit

www.lowkcalgal.com/journal.

and grab your free journal now.

About the Author

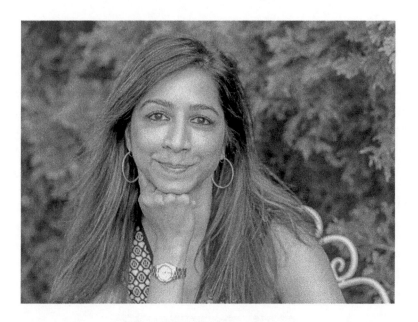

S ameera Khan is a bariatric dietitian and physician's assistant in the field of bariatrics. She specializes in helping weight loss surgery patients reach their weight loss goals and prevent weight regain. With a bachelors in nutrition, graduate studies as a physician assistant, along with a degree in health care management, Sameera also teaches nutrition at a local community college. She sees firsthand what the life of a bariatric patient looks like. She works with them to help them create a life that they will love years after bariatric surgery.

Sameera has been privileged to be trained and mentored by some of the most noted bariatric surgeons in the industry. She has utilized her knowledge and skills in her coordinator role for many years to help bariatric patients during their maintenance phase. Sameera is excited to bring her skills and expertise on weight regain after bariatric surgery to the public world with her guidance, weight loss retreats, and monthly weight loss-in-a-box subscriptions. Sameera reminds us that bariatric surgery is not a miracle but a "tool" that you need to keep well-oiled and working in specific and deliberate ways. This isn't just a theory but the result-based product of real-life bariatric patients you meet in this book. If it worked for them, get ready to make it work for you!

Sameera inspires audiences to open doors and achieve success in their weight loss journeys and their lives. Her expertise in working with bariatric patients will encourage the reader to understand and manage weight regain by getting out of the "no" mode and start living in the "yes" mode.

Her passion of helping others has motivated her to create an innovative concept and practical system that changes how to handle the weight regain response which she has learned through her extensive research and unique approach. The lasting results will lead to a healthier, more productive life for all bariatric surgery patients.

She helps people break free from the weight loss cycle they are in. Losing weight should not be a lifelong event and yet many people face that exact situation for most of their lives even after bariatric surgery. Always trying and always failing, making losing weight a hopeless battle. Not anymore.

This resource streamlines the reasons for weight regain after bariatric surgery and how to gain control over the transformation processes down into simple, straightforward, actionable strategies, and step-by-step guides.

Most of the weight loss industry focuses on selling people a bunch of gimmicky diets that they don't really need, like "get fit quick" schemes, or processed meal subscriptions that work temporarily.

Sameera's approach is different. Her mission is to blend her formal education in obesity studies, with almost two decades of experience as a weight loss dietitian. A successful coordinator, coach, and guide, it is her passion to help patients reach their goals in the most effective, efficient, and sustainable ways possible.

Bibliography

Ahmed, Kasim, et al. "Taste Changes after Bariatric Surgery: a Systematic Review." *Obesity Surgery*, vol. 28, no. 10, 2018, pp. 3321–3332., doi:10.1007/s11695-018-3420-8.

Al-Najim, Werd, Neil G. Docherty, and Carel W. Le Roux. "Food Intake and Eating Behavior After Bariatric Surgery." *Physiological Reviews* 98, no. 3 (2018): 1113-1141. doi:10.1152/physrev.00021.2017.

Avena, Nicole M, and Mark S Gold. "Variety and Hyperpalatability: Are They Promoting Addictive Overeating?" *The American Journal of Clinical Nutrition*, vol. 94, no. 2, 2011, pp. 367–368., doi:10.3945/ajcn.111.020164.

Bradberry, Travis, and Jean Greaves. *Emotional Intelligence 2.0.* San Diego, CA: TalentSmart, 2009.

Brandão, Isabel, et al. "A Psychiatric Perspective View of Bariatric Surgery Patients." *Archives of Clinical Psychiatry (São Paulo)*, vol. 42, no. 5, 2015, pp. 122–128., doi:10.1590/0101-60830000000062

Burke, Lora E., Jing Wang, and Mary Ann Sevick. "Self-Monitoring in Weight Loss: A Systematic Review of the Literature." *Journal of the American Dietetic Association* 111, no. 1 (2011): 92-102. doi:10.1016/j.jada.2010.10.008

Chen, Jung-Chien, et al. "Effect of Probiotics on Postoperative Quality of Gastric Bypass Surgeries: a Prospective Randomized Trial." *Surgery for Obesity and Related Diseases*, vol. 12, no. 1, 2016, pp. 57–61., doi:10.1016/j.soard.2015.07.010.

Chou, Wen-Ying Sylvia, et al. "Obesity in Social Media: a Mixed Methods Analysis." *Translational Behavioral Medicine*, vol. 4, no. 3, 2014, pp. 314–323., doi:10.1007/s13142-014-0256-1.

Cohen, Bruce H., Dr. Comment on "Mitochondrial Myopathy with Dr. Bruce Cohen." *Mitochondrial Myopathy* (audio blog). Accessed May 3, 2019. http://www.mitoaction.org/podcasts/mitochondrial-myopathy-dr-bruce-cohen.

Cordeiro, Felicia, et al. "Barriers and Negative Nudges." *Proceedings of the 33rd Annual ACM Conference on Human Factors in Computing Systems - CHI '15*, 2015, doi:10.1145/2702123.2702155.

Calories Burned Dancing Calculator. Captain Calculator, 2014, captaincalculator.com/health/calorie/calories-burned-dancing-calculator/.

Drewnowski, Adam, et al. "Sugar and Fat: Sensory and Hedonic Evaluation of Liquid and Solid Foods." *Physiology & Behavior*, vol. 45, no. 1, 1989, pp. 177–183., doi:10.1016/0031-9384(89)90182-0.

Ekmekcioglu, Cem, et al. "Salt Taste after Bariatric Surgery and Weight Loss in Obese Persons." *PeerJ*, vol. 4, 2016, doi:10.7717/peerj.2086.

El-Hadi, Mustafa, et al. "The Effect of Bariatric Surgery on Gastroesophageal Reflux Disease." *Canadian Journal of Surgery*, vol. 57, no. 2, 2014, pp. 139–144., doi:10.1503/cjs.030612.

Farias, Maria Magdalena, et al. "Set-Point Theory and Obesity." *Metabolic Syndrome and Related Disorders*, vol. 9, no. 2, 2011, pp. 85–89., doi:10.1089/met.2010.0090.

Fernström, Maria, Linda Bakkman, Peter Loogna, Olav Rooyackers, Madeleine Svensson, Towe Jakobsson, Lena Brandt, and Ylva Trolle Lagerros. "Improved Muscle Mitochondrial Capacity Following Gastric Bypass Surgery in Obese Subjects." *Obesity Surgery* 26, no. 7 (2015): 1391-397. doi:10.1007/s11695-015-1932-z.

Fotuhi O, Fong GT, Zanna MP, Borland R, Yong HH, Cummings KM. Patterns , *Journal of Experimental Social Psychology* 51 (2014). doi:10.1016/s0022-1031(13)00212-6.

Framson, Celia, Alan R. Kristal, Jeannette M. Schenk, Alyson J. Littman, Steve Zeliadt, and Denise Benitez. "Development and Validation of the Mindful Eating Questionnaire." *Journal of the American Dietetic Association* 109, no. 8 (2009): 1439-444. doi:10.1016/j.jada.2009.05.006

Gearhardt, Ashley N., et al. "The Addiction Potential of Hyperpalatable Foods." *Current Drug Abuse Reviewse*, vol. 4, no. 3, 2011, pp. 140–145., doi:10.2174/1874473711104030140

Gottfried, Sara. *"The Hormone Reset Diet: Heal Your Metabolism to Lose up to 15 Pounds in 21 Days*. Toronto: Collins, 2017

Gundry, Steve. *The Plant Paradox: The Hidden Dangers in "healthy" Foods That Cause Disease and Weight Gain*. New York, NY: Harper Collins, 2017

Guo, Yan, et al. "Modulation of the Gut Microbiome: a Systematic Review of the Effect of Bariatric Surgery." *European Journal of Endocrinology*, vol. 178, no. 1, 2018, pp. 43–56., doi:10.1530/eje-17-0403.

Haluzík, Martin, and Miloš Mráz. "Intermittent Fasting and Prevention of Diabetic Retinopathy: Where Do We Go From Here?" *Diabetes*, vol. 67, no. 9,
2018, pp. 1745–1747., doi:10.2337/dbi18-0022

Harris, Leanne, et al. "Intermittent Fasting Interventions for Treatment of Overweight and Obesity in Adults." *JBI Database of Systematic Reviews and
Implementation Reports*, vol. 16, no. 2, 2018, pp. 507–547., doi:10.11124/
jbisrir-2016-003248.

Health, Omada. "The Omada Program." Omada. Accessed April 26, 2019.
https://go.omadahealth.com/.

"Heart Rate Calculator." *The Skinny on Health, Fitness, and Weight Loss*,
2019, www.superskinnyme.com/heart-rate-calculator.html.sk

Hill, James O., et al. "Using the Energy Gap to Address Obesity: A Commen-
tary." *Journal of the American Dietetic Association*, vol. 109, no. 11, 2009,
pp. 1848–1853., doi:10.1016/j.jada.2009.08.007.

Ho-Pham, Lan T., et al. "More on Body Fat Cutoff Points." *Mayo Clinic Proceedings*, vol. 86, no. 6, 2011, p. 584., doi:10.4065/mcp.2011.0097.

Ic, De S Porcelli. "Effects of Bariatric Surgery on the Oral Health of Patients."
International Journal of Dentistry and Oral Health 2, no. 2 (2016).
doi:10.16966/2378-7090.181.

Jackson, Chandra L., and Frank B. Hu. "Long-term Associations of Nut Consumption with Body Weight and Obesity." *The American Journal of Clinical Nutrition* 100, no. Suppl_1 (2014). doi:10.3945/ajcn.113.071332

Jumbe, Sandra, et al. "The Effectiveness of Bariatric Surgery on Long Term
Psychosocial Quality of Life – A Systematic Review." *Obesity Research
& Clinical Practice*, vol. 10, no. 3, 2016, pp. 225–242., doi:10.1016/j.
orcp.2015.11.009.

Kabat-Zinn, Jon. *Wherever You Go, There You Are: Mindfulness Meditation in
Everyday Life*. Hyperion, 1994.

Kechagia, Maria, et al. "Health Benefits of Probiotics: A Review." *ISRN Nutrition*, vol. 2013, 2013, pp. 1–7., doi:10.5402/2013/481651.

Koball, Afton M., et al. "Content and Accuracy of Nutrition-Related Posts in
Bariatric Surgery Facebook Support Groups." *Surgery for Obesity and
Related Diseases*, vol. 14, no. 12, 2018, pp. 1897–1902., doi:10.1016/j.
soard.2018.08.017.

Komaroff, Anthony. "Major Fat-burning Discovery." *Harvard Health Publishing*, June 2012.

Knäuper, Bärbel, Rowena Pillay, Julien Lacaille, Amanda Mccollam, and
Evan Kelso. "Replacing Craving Imagery with Alternative Pleasant

Imagery Reduces Craving Intensity." *Appetite* 57, no. 1 (2011): 173-78. doi:10.1016/j.appet.2011.04.021.

Lanza, Ian R. "Enhancing the Metabolic Benefits of Bariatric Surgery: Tipping the Scales With Exercise: Figure 1." *Diabetes*, vol. 64, no. 11, 2015, pp. 3656–3658., doi:10.2337/dbi15-0018.

Leahey, Tricia M., et al. "Effects of Bariatric Surgery on Food Cravings: Do Food Cravings and the Consumption of Craved Foods 'Normalize' after Surgery?" *Surgery for Obesity and Related Diseases*, vol. 8, no. 1, 2012, pp. 84–91., doi:10.1016/j.soard.2011.07.016.

Levine, James A., Mark W. Vander Weg, James O. Hill, and Robert C. Klesges. "Non-Exercise Activity Thermogenesis." *Arteriosclerosis, Thrombosis, and Vascular Biology* 26, no. 4 (2006): 729-36. doi:10.1161/01. atv.0000205848.83210.73.

Liangpunsakul, Suthat, David W. Crabb, and Rong Qi. "Relationship Among Alcohol Intake, Body Fat, and Physical Activity: A Population-Based Study." *Annals of Epidemiology* 20, no. 9 (2010): 670-75. doi:10.1016/j. annepidem.2010.05.014.

Lipski, Elizabeth. *Digestive Wellness: Strengthen the Immune System and Prevent Disease through Healthy Digestion*. New York, NY: McGraw-Hill, 2012.

Ludwig, David. *Always Hungry?: Conquer Cravings, Retrain Your Fat Cells, and Lose Weight Permanently*. New York: Grand Central Life & Style, 2018.

Ludwig, David. *Always Hungry?: Conquer Cravings, Retrain Your Fat Cells, and Lose Weight Permanently*. Grand Central Life & Style, 2018.

Ma, Yu, et al. "Dietary Fiber Intake and Risks of Proximal and Distal Colon Cancers." *Medicine*, vol. 97, no. 36, 2018, doi:10.1097/md.0000000000011678

Madsbad, Sten, et al. "Mechanisms of Changes in Glucose Metabolism and Bodyweight after Bariatric Surgery." *The Lancet Diabetes & Endocrinology*, vol. 2, no. 2, 2014, pp. 152–164., doi:10.1016/s2213-8587(13)70218-3.

Major, Piotr, et al. "Quality of Life After Bariatric Surgery." *Obesity Surgery*, vol. 25, no. 9, 2015, pp. 1703–1710., doi:10.1007/s11695-015-1601-2.

Nakajima, Atsushi, et al. "Safety and Efficacy of Elobixibat for Chronic Constipation: Results from a Randomized, Double-Blind, Placebo-Controlled, Phase 3 Trial and an Open-Label, Single-Arm, Phase 3 Trial." *The Lancet Gastroenterology & Hepatology*, vol. 3, no. 8, 2018, pp. 537–547., doi:10.1016/s2468-1253(18)30123-7

National Institute on Alcohol Abuse and Alcoholism. Accessed May 03, 2019. http:// www.rethinkingdrinking.niaaa.nih.gov/tools/calculators/calorie-calculator.aspx

Nauert, Rick. "Brain Scans Show Cognitive Benefits of Exercise Over Time." *Psych Central*, March 27, 2019.

https://psychcentral.com/news/2019/03/27/brain-scans-show-cognitive-benefits-of-exercise-over-time/144097.html

Paoli, Antonio. "Ketogenic Diet for Obesity: Friend or Foe?" *International Journal of Environmental Research and Public Health*, vol. 11, no. 2, 2014, pp. 2092–2107., doi:10.3390/ijerph110202092.

Peeke, Pamela. "Dr Pamela Peeke on Food Addiction, "Fat Genes," and the Three M's." Accessed May 3, 2019. https://tipsofthescale.com/51-dr-pamela-peeke/.

Phillips, Katherine M., et al. "Phytosterol Composition of Nuts and Seeds Commonly Consumed in the United States." *Journal of Agricultural and Food Chemistry*, vol. 53, no. 24, 2005, pp. 9436–9445., doi:10.1021/jf051505h.

Richardson, W. S., A.M Plaisance, L. Periou, J. Buquoi, and D. Tillery. "Long-term Management of Patients after Weight Loss Surgery." *The Ochsner Journal* 9 (2009): 154-59.

Spalding, Kirsty L., Erik Arner, Pål O. Westermark, Samuel Bernard, Bruce A. Buchholz, Olaf Bergmann, Lennart Blomqvist, Johan Hoffstedt, Erik Näslund, Tom Britton, Hernan Concha, Moustapha Hassan, Mikael Rydén, Jonas Frisén, and Peter Arner. "Dynamics of Fat Cell Turnover in Humans." *Nature* 453, no. 7196 (2008): 783-87. doi:10.1038/nature06902.

Stillwell, David. "Obesity Complicates Dental Health." *Obesity Action Coalition*. https://www.obesityaction.org/community/article.../obesity-complicates-dental-health/

Swift, Kathie Madonna, Joseph Hooper, and Mark Hyman. *The Swift Diet: 4 Weeks to Mend the Belly, Lose the Weight, and Get Rid of the Bloat*. NY, NY: Plume, 2015

Thornton, Simon N. "Increased Hydration Can Be Associated with Weight Loss." *Frontiers in Nutrition*, vol. 3, 2016, doi:10.3389/fnut.2016.00018.

Tofighi, B., A. Abrantes, and M.D Stein. "The Role of Technology Based Interventions for Substance Abuse Disorders in Primary Care: A Review of the Literature." *Med Clin North America* 102, no. 4 (2018): 715-31.

Vetter, Celine, and Frank A.j. l. Scheer. "Circadian Biology: Uncoupling Human Body Clocks by Food Timing." *Current Biology*, vol. 27, no. 13, 2017, doi:10.1016/j.cub.2017.05.057

Wahls, Terry MD: "Mitochondria, Health & Vegetables." Interview. *Mitochondria, Health & Vegetables* (audio blog). Accessed May 3, 2019. https://blog.bulletproof.com/120-dr-terry-wahls-on-mitochondria-health-and-vegetables-podcast/.

Wansink, B. (2006). Mindless Eating: Why We Eat More Than We Think. *New York: Bantam Books*.

Wansink, Brian, and Jeffery Sobal. "Mindless Eating." *Environment and Behavior*, vol. 39, no. 1, 2007, pp. 106–123., doi:10.1177/0013916506295573.

Wilkens, Carrie. "What's the First Step of Habit Change? Going off Autopilot!" *Coping with Urges* (blog). Accessed May 3, 2019. https://www.smartrecovery.org/tag/carrie-wilkens/.

Wimmelmann, Cathrine L., et al. "Psychological Predictors of Weight Loss after Bariatric Surgery: A Review of the Recent Research." *Obesity Research & Clinical Practice*, vol. 8, no. 4, 2014, doi:10.1016/j.orcp.2013.09.003.

Yoder, Ruth, et al. "How Do Individuals Develop Alcohol Use Disorder After Bariatric Surgery? A Grounded Theory Exploration." *Obesity Surgery*, vol. 28, no. 3, 2017, pp. 717–724., doi:10.1007/s11695-017-2936-7.

Printed in the USA
CPSIA information can be obtained
at www.ICGtesting.com
JSHW082229140824
68134JS00017B/805